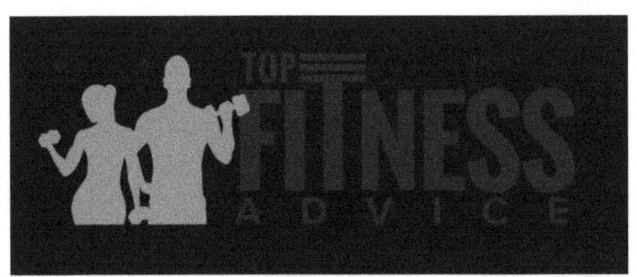

ULTIMATE KETOSIS GUIDE

The 100 Day Ketogenic Diet That Will COMPLETELY Transform Your Body!

(BONUS: 150+ Keto Diet Recipes)

Kayla Bates

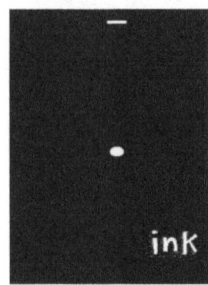

First published in 2017 by Venture Ink Publishing

Copyright © Top Fitness Advice 2019

All rights reserved.

No part of this book may be reproduced in any form without permission in writing from the author. No part of this publication may be reproduced or transmitted in any form or by any means, mechanic, electronic, photocopying, recording, by any storage or retrieval system, or transmitted by email without the permission in writing from the author and publisher.

Requests to the publisher for permission should be addressed to publishing@ventureink.co

For more information about the contents of this book or questions to the author, please contact Kayla Bates at kayla@topfitnessadvice.com

Disclaimer

This book provides wellness management information in an informative and educational manner only, with information that is general in nature and that is not specific to you, the reader. The contents of this book are intended to assist you and other readers in your personal wellness efforts. Consult your physician regarding the applicability of any information provided in this book to you.

Nothing in this book should be construed as personal advice or diagnosis, and must not be used in this manner. The information provided about conditions is general in nature. This information does not cover all possible uses, actions, precautions, side-effects, or interactions of medicines, or medical procedures. The information in this book should not be considered as complete and does not cover all diseases, ailments, physical conditions, or their treatment.

You should consult with your physician before beginning any exercise, weight loss, or health care program. This book should not be used in place of a call or visit to a competent health-care professional. You should consult a health care professional before adopting any of the suggestions in this book or before drawing inferences from it.

Any decision regarding treatment and medication for your condition should be made with the advice and consultation of a qualified health care professional. If you have, or suspect you have, a health-care problem, then you should immediately contact a qualified health care professional for treatment.

No Warranties: The author and publisher don't guarantee or warrant the quality, accuracy, completeness, timeliness, appropriateness or suitability of the information in this book, or of any product or services referenced in this book.

The information in this book is provided on an "as is" basis and the author and publisher make no representations or warranties of any kind with respect to this information. This book may contain inaccuracies, typographical errors, or other errors.

Liability Disclaimer: The publisher, author, and other parties involved in the creation, production, provision of information, or delivery of this book specifically disclaim any responsibility, and shall not be held liable for any damages, claims, injuries, losses, liabilities, costs, or obligations including any direct, indirect, special, incidental, or consequences damages (collectively known as "Damages") whatsoever and howsoever caused, arising out of, or in connection with the use or misuse of the site and the information contained within it, whether such Damages arise in contract, tort, negligence, equity, statute law, or by way of other legal theory.

Table of Contents

Disclaimer	3
Who Is This Book For?	7
What Will This Book Teach You?	8
Introduction	9
Chapter 1: Why Should You Go on A Ketogenic Diet?	11
Chapter 2: Effects of the Ketogenic Diet	16
Chapter 3: Getting Started with the Ketogenic Diet	21
Chapter 4: Ketogenic Diet Plan	33
Chapter 5: Low-Carb Living Tips for Weight Loss	43
Chapter 6: Tips for Success on the Ketogenic Diet	46
Chapter 7: Low-Carb Diet Myths Debunked	48
Chapter 8: Ketogenic Diet Recipes	52
Conclusion	278
Final Words	279

Would you prefer to listen to my book, rather than read it?

Download the audiobook version for free!

If you go to the special link below and sign up to Audible as a new customer, you can get the audiobook version of my book completely free.

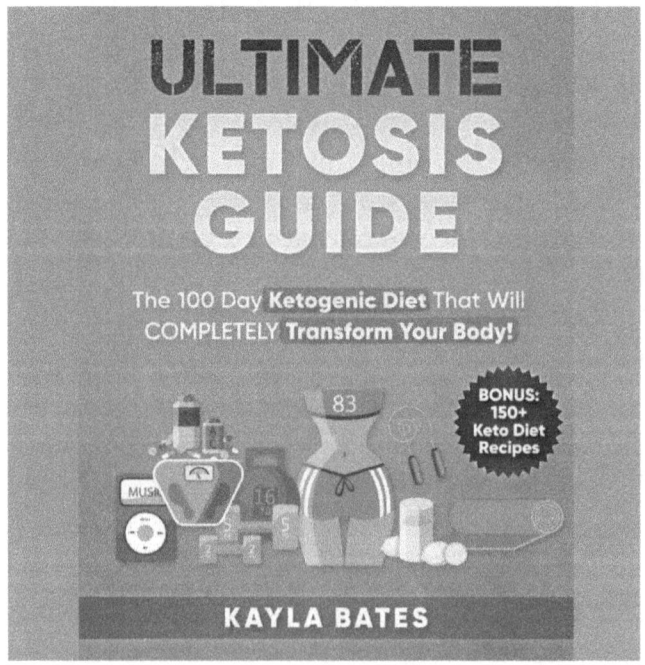

Go here to get your audiobook version for free:

TopFitnessAdvice.com/go/UltimateKetosis

Who Is This Book For?

This eye-opening book is simply for those who are gaining weight terribly and they are ready to transform their bodies completely using the ketogenic diet.

Maybe it took you years of slow weight gain to reach your current weight – reverting to your previous lifestyle will result in a gradual return to this burden. If you do not achieve the knowledge you need to keep weight off, then weight loss will forever be a rollercoaster.

There will be periods in your life when you are at your ideal weight, and those years will be full of fun and joy, but eventually that pressure will return unless you follow this guide "THE 100 DAY KETOGENIC DIET THAT WILL COMPLETELY TRANSFORM YOUR BODY PLUS 150 KETO DIET RECIPES"

Many guides are going to offer advice and suggestions on what you can do to lose weight, but many of them are unsafe, offer bad advice, and are just too hard to follow for the long term.

This book is second to one and my advice to you is that you read through this ketosis guide and act immediately I am sure it will help transform your body completely.

What Will This Book Teach You?

This ketosis guide explores how to make the ketogenic diet work the best for your weight loss needs. It brings up the important issue of weight loss by explaining how to get started with the ketogenic diet and how to follow the ketogenic diet plan precisely.

It again explains the tips and tricks to get the most out of the ketogenic diet and the ketogenic diet recipes. Through the benefits of ketogenic diet outlined in the book you will be motivated to use this method for amazing results.

This guide teaches you many things including the ways to take your intermittent fasting to the next level and how the whole process works. It also outlines the low carb diet myths, you can try new things, and stay focused.

Read through this guide and bet me you will contact me and share the success news.

Introduction

Firstly, the word ketosis refers to the state of the human body when it lacks carbohydrates and starts depending upon proteins, fat, and muscle for its energy. That is how this diet got its name. In other words, a ketosis diet is a diet with a few carbs or no carbs at all.

Being in this condition, the brain tells your body to create reserves of glucose for emergencies only. It happens because of the lack of carbohydrates in your body. And so, the brain starts using fat storages for immediate energy needs.

Ketosis is the second part of the process that takes place when your body's metabolism shifts from getting energy from carbohydrates to taking it from fat. When it is taking place, this is the time you lose the fattest.

The term ketosis relates to the blocks of fat that are stored for release as energy, which is known as ketones. Thank you for purchasing this book it is my sincere hope that it will answer all your questions on the ketogenic diet.

Are You ALWAYS Hungry When You Try to Lose Weight?

Discover How to STOP Starving Yourself & Lose Weight FASTER By Eating MORE Food!

For this month only, you can get Kayla's best-selling & most popular book absolutely free – *The Ultimate Guide to Healthy Eating & Losing Weight Without Starving Yourself!*

Get Your FREE Copy Here:

TopFitnessAdvice.com/Book

Discover how you can **start eating MORE food** and see weight loss results faster than ever before. Learn about the 10 most powerful fat-burning foods and how they boost the rate that your body burns fat. And last but not least, finally put an end to your emotional or "bored" eating habits. With this book, readers were able to significantly improve their weight loss results. So, it's highly recommended that you get this book, especially while it's free!

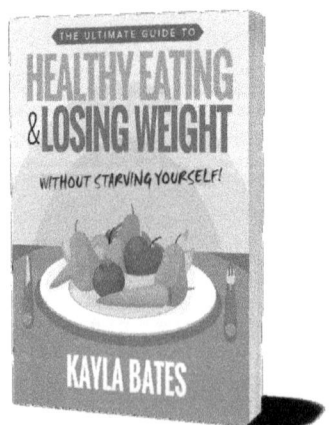

Get Your FREE Copy Here:

TopFitnessAdvice.com/Book

Chapter 1

Why Should You Go on A Ketogenic Diet?

The truth is that the ketogenic diet has always been controversial. Many people have condemned the food but the question the critics have been unable to provide a clear answer to is "Why is a diet that is highly recommended for treatment of various illnesses so demonic for weight loss?"

The ketogenic diet most certainly comes with its set of drawbacks (which food, health procedure or treatment doesn't?) but the truth is that the health benefits of the ketogenic diet exceed its disadvantages.

Some of the proven health benefits of the ketogenic diet include:

- **Curbs Your Appetite**

    You will agree with me that if you can find a way to reduce your appetite, your battle against excess weight gain is half won. Also, most people are unable to follow through with any diet plan that enables them to lose weight because they fail to control the hunger.

    The ketogenic diet, however, helps you to curb your appetite and makes you feel less hungry because of the increased consumption of fat and proteins, which fills you up for much longer.

- **Increased Weight Loss**

    The fastest way to lose weight without starving yourself is to cut back on carbohydrates.

- **Helps with Abdominal Fat Loss**

If you've been struggling with weight loss for some time now, you would know that abdominal fat is the most difficult type of fat to get rid of.

Sometimes, people lose weight in other areas of their body but are still unable to lose the fat in their stomach because the type of fat that is stored in the abdomen is visceral fat, a very stubborn type of fat. Well, the good news is that low carbohydrate diets like the ketogenic diet are very useful for getting rid of abdominal fat.

- **Reduces Triglycerides**

Triglycerides are fat molecules present in the body, and they are a very well-known risk factor for heart diseases. Low carb diets such as the ketogenic diet can reduce triglycerides in the blood and prevent heart diseases caused by excessive triglycerides in the body.

- **Increases HDL Levels**

High-Density Lipoprotein, also known as HDL is a type of lipoprotein that helps to carry cholesterol around the body. It is nicknamed the 'good cholesterol' as it is a better version than the Low-Density Lipoprotein LDL known as the 'bad cholesterol.'

Increased HDL levels in the body help to ensure that cholesterol is eliminated from the body by transporting it to the liver for reuse or excretion. It is unlike the LDL, which carries the cholesterol from the liver back into the body. Consuming a lot of healthy fats as is done on the Ketogenic diet, helps to increase HDL levels in the body.

- **Reduces Blood Sugar Levels**

People who have Type 2 diabetes can also benefit from the ketogenic diet as it helps to lower blood sugar and insulin concentrations in the body. When you consume carbohydrates, what your body does is to break it down into glucose in your digestive tract then the glucose goes into your bloodstream and causes your blood sugar levels to increase.

This increase in blood sugar levels is very harmful to your body, so your body tries to protect itself by producing the insulin hormone to burn or store the excess glucose. People who do not suffer from insulin resistance problems can get their blood glucose levels reduced quickly.

However, many people suffer from insulin resistance, which makes it difficult for their cells to respond to insulin. It makes it difficult for blood glucose levels to be reduced in the body and eventually leads to what is known as type 2 diabetes.

The good news is that the consumption of a low-carbohydrate diet can, however, help the body with eliminating excess blood glucose without the aid of insulin.

- **Reduces Blood Pressure**

    The Ketogenic diet may also help with reducing blood pressure and prevent blood pressure related diseases like stroke, kidney problems, and heart problem.

- **Helps with Treating Metabolic Syndrome**

    Metabolic syndrome is a condition that causes some other circumstances in the body such as an increase in blood pressure, high blood sugar levels, excess body fat and abdominal fat and high triglycerides. These conditions may increase a person's risk of suffering from diabetes, stroke and other heart-related diseases.

A Ketogenic diet can help to help people suffering from metabolic syndrome significantly.

- **Helps with Treating Brain Disorders**

    Low carbohydrate diets can also help with treating brain disorders such as Alzheimer's disease and Parkinson disease.

Just like many things in life, the Ketogenic diet also has its set of drawbacks that we will discuss briefly in the next chapter.

Benefits of the Ketogenic Diet

The list of advantages concerning a ketogenic diet is a lengthy and happy one. These are some of the perks of the food you can expect to see after a month of switching to the ketogenic diet plan:

Being in ketosis allows the body to process fat and use it as fuel.

Another benefit of being in a state of ketosis is that excess ketone are not harmful to your system in any way whatsoever.

Insulin is one of the substances that make you crave food, particularly because it is high in sugar, and so controlling it at healthy levels is one of the key elements of weight loss.

Most research studies on the benefits of ketosis diets for epileptic seizures in children show a large improvement, which is especially significant since these kids usually did not respond to previous medication therapy.

Last, but certainly not least, is that a majority of people who take advantage of ketogenic diet weight loss when you're not fighting cravings and hunger every step of the way. In fact, hunger pangs can often derail a person's best efforts! Not having to deal with them makes it easier to meet your goals, all the way around.

Drawbacks

As I mentioned earlier, the Ketogenic diet is not rid of its set of drawbacks. Some of the challenges of the ketogenic diets include:

1. **Low-Energy Levels**: People who work in jobs that require high levels of energy or athletes may face challenges on starting the ketogenic diet because of the reduced energy levels.

2. **Restrictive Eating**: You can't eat whatever you please on this diet as there are rules. That's why many people find it difficult to cope with such high levels of eating discipline.

3. **Metabolic Problems**: Critics also believe that going on a low-carbohydrate diet for an extended period may upset normal metabolic function.

Some people also tend to overdo the low carb thing. They cut away essential things like fruits and vegetables that are beneficial for the body and end up depriving their bodies of essential nutrients and vitamins. It is why it is imperative for you to do an extensive and proper research on the ketogenic diet before embarking on it so that you can do it right and avoid these problems.

Chapter 2

Effects of the Ketogenic Diet

How the Body Utilizes Various Fuels

In the human body, there are three primary storage 'depots' of fuel that can be tapped into for supply of energy when there is a caloric deficiency.

- The body would tap into its protein storage and convert it to glucose in the liver

- The body can tap into its carbohydrate (glycogen) store

- The body can as well make use of its fat storage, which is stored in the body as body fat.

There is also a fourth type of fuel, which the body can use known as ketones. On a typical diet, the ketones are insignificant to the body for energy production. However, on a low-carbohydrate diet such as the ketogenic diet, ketones are used a lot as a source of energy, especially by the brain.

Body tissues always make use of the most available source of fuel in the bloodstream. For instance, if there is a high concentration of glucose in the body, the body chooses glucose as its most preferred source of fuel except for organs like the heart that make use of a mixture of glucose, ketones and free fatty acids for fuel.

If, however, there is a reduction of the concentration of glucose in the body, the body will have to choose the next available source of fuel as its source of energy. On a ketogenic diet, the body switches from using glucose as its primary source of fuel to making use of stored fats due to the increased availability of fats in the body.

One of the goals of a ketogenic diet, therefore, is to increase the concentration of proteins and fats in the body as opposed to carbohydrate so that the body can switch to burning fat for energy to also burn the excess fat stored in the body.

There are however some other factors apart from fuel concentration, which contribute to determining which fuels will be used by the body. They include levels of insulin and glucagon hormones in the body and levels of regulatory enzymes for breakdown of glucose and fats.

Ketone Bodies and Ketogenesis

There are three known types of ketone bodies namely Acetoacetate, Beta-hydroxybutyrate, and Acetone. The process by which these ketones are formed is what is known as ketogenesis, and to understand the ketogenic diet, it is important for you to grasp the concept of ketogenesis fully. Ketogenesis in the body depends on two major factors; the liver and the fat cells.

Fat Cells

Breakdown of fat cells in the body is dependent on the catecholamines and the insulin hormones. When there are high levels of insulin in the blood, it prevents mobilization of free fatty acids and increases fat storage in the body through the lipoprotein lipase enzyme (LPL).

As insulin levels in the blood reduce, mobilization of free fatty acids improve. It travels through the bloodstream aided by a protein known as Albumin, and then when it is in the blood, it can be used for energy production. Free fatty acids that are not used as fuel would be oxidized in the liver.

This oxidization leads to the production of ketone bodies, which are then released back into the bloodstream.

Liver

Along with the fat cells, the liver is another imperative factor that determines ketogenesis in the body. The liver always produces ketones, whether on a ketogenic diet or not but in small and hardly significant quantities.

The ketogenic diet, however, increases amounts of ketones present in the body. So, when people tell you ketones are harmful byproducts, remind them that ketones are always present in the body.

The liver is very essential for ketogenesis because even if there are high levels of free fatty acids in the body, there would be no production of ketones if the liver is not in a ketogenic 'mood.'

What determines whether the liver would produce ketone bodies or otherwise is the amount of liver glycogen available.

The liver glycogen's primary function is to help maintain healthy glucose levels. So, when you are on a low carb diet, and the blood glucose levels are reduced, the liver glycogen prompts the liver to break down its glycogen stores and release glucose into the bloodstream.

Your body makes use of this glucose for some time (between 12 and 16 hours depending on levels of physical activities), after which its glycogen stores become depleted. Upon depletion, ketogenesis increases rapidly according to the availability of free fatty acids.

Metabolic Effects of the Ketogenic Diet

One thing that critics are always quick to shout when the ketogenic diet is mentioned is that "the ketogenic diet will mess up your metabolism."

So, will the ketogenic diet mess up your metabolism?

What your metabolic system primarily does is to make fuels available in your body whenever they are needed. As you continue to consume foods, your metabolic system continues to work to ensure that the energy from the foods are appropriately allocated, and then the excesses are stored.

The average human today eats too much, and as a result, the metabolic system has to cope with more work than it is designed to handle.

During the starvation diet, the metabolic system focuses on the provision of glucose for tissues that necessarily require glucose to function such as the brain, kidney, red blood cells, etc. This glucose is usually gotten from the body's protein stores; mainly the muscles and sometimes from fat.

Your metabolic system doesn't know how long this starvation is going to continue; maybe for a few hours or some few weeks?

It first tries to cope with the situation by plundering the glucose supply in the blood and then takes some proteins from the muscles.

But because it must also ensure that muscle mass is not excessively depleted, it turns to the ketones for a solution.

Ketones can stand in for glucose and proteins so the muscles are spared from depletion, and your body is happy with using its new-found source of fuel; ketones for energy.

This is what happens on a starvation diet but a low carb diet; you would be eating some proteins and fats, so your muscles need not be depleted; the proteins you consume are converted to glucose.

So, will this diet ruin your metabolism?

First, you must understand that metabolism is not just dependent on what you eat but on some other factors including Basal metabolic rate, thermic effect of food and physical activity.

Basal Metabolic Rate: Your basal metabolic rate, for instance, is dependent on the amount of lean body mass you have, your hormonal homeostasis, genetic tendencies and your present body fat levels amongst other factors.

All diets, including normal dietary conditions, would affect the basal metabolic rate and the hormonal outcome, and body composition of weight loss is what affects your metabolic rate and not just the type of diet you follow.

Thermic Effect of Food: This energy breaks down the macronutrients from consumed foods and processes them. Protein makes use of the highest amount of energy to be given out. This is why low-carb diets improve metabolism, but the same thing would happen on any diet that increases consumption of protein and not just the ketogenic diet.

Thermic Effect of Activity: This refers to any form of activity that is not a necessary body function such as exercises. People who are physically inactive and live sedentary lifestyles may only burn 10-30 percent more calories over their BMR, but physically active individuals who use regularly would consume more.

So you see, it's not only what you eat that affects your metabolism; as long as you maintain a moderate level of physical activity and avoid complete starvation, you would be able to maintain a healthy metabolism.

What Not to Expect from the Ketogenic Diet: The diet is not a miracle weight loss solution or a yo-yo diet. It is a lifestyle change that takes a lot of discipline and hard work on your part to make it work. However, once you get used to the rudiments of the diet, you would begin to enjoy it and lose the weight very quickly.

You shouldn't also expect this diet to work without exercise. For better weight loss results, you should do the ketogenic diet along with regular exercise.

Chapter 3

Getting Started with the Ketogenic Diet

Now that you have all the necessary information about the ketogenic diet; what it entails and how it works, it's time to move to the primary purpose of this book how to do the ketogenic diet.

There are various variations of the ketogenic diet as you would see below.

However, before we go on to discuss the different versions of the ketogenic diet, you must first measure your nutritional needs on a ketogenic diet. It would give you an idea of what your minimum caloric intake daily should be based on how much calories your body burns daily.

You can make use of this online keto calculator to quickly determine that.

Different Variations of the Ketogenic Diet

1. **The Standard Ketogenic Diet**

    It is the original version of the diet used as far as the late 1800's and the early 1900's as a remedy for pediatric epilepsy. It involves consuming low amounts of carbohydrates with moderate amounts of protein and high amounts of fats.

    On the standard ketogenic diet, there is a high level of carbohydrate restriction with about 20 -50 grams or less recommended daily to induce ketosis.

    Fruits and starches are to be avoided entirely on the standard ketogenic diet, but you can consume carbohydrates from green leafy vegetables because they have a very low glycemic index and less effect on insulin release.

2. **The Targeted Ketogenic Diet**

   Due to the restrictions of the standard ketogenic diet, the targeted ketogenic diet was developed for physically active people (like people who work jobs that require physical agility).

   On the targeted ketogenic diet, carbs are to be consumed around workout times (30-60 minutes before workout) so as to maintain physical performance and allow glycogen re-synthesis without affecting ketosis while at other occasions, a low carb, moderate to high protein and fat diet should be kept.

3. **The Cyclical Ketogenic Diet**

   Bodybuilders, weightlifters, and athletes require a lot of energy for performance. This power may exceed what they may not get when on the standard ketogenic diet. So, the cyclical ketogenic diet was developed to cater to their ketogenic needs.

   On the cyclical ketogenic diet, you would be required to alternate between periods of high carb consumption and years of low carb consumption to increase weight loss and sustain energy for exercise. You would be required to do between 5 to 6 days of low carb ketogenic dieting and alternate that with 1-2 days of high carb consumption. You may also do longer cycles; 12-13 days of low carb consumption and 2-3 days of high carb consumption.

Dieting Principles

Doing the ketogenic diet requires adhering to some principles which include the following:

- 60-75% of your daily calories should come from fat, 15-30% from protein and only 5-10% should come from carbohydrates.

- Your daily net carbs consumption should be less than 50 grams. Daily net carbs are calculated by deducting fiber contents from carbohydrate contents.

- Eat moderate amounts of proteins. You can use your body fat percentage to determine the most appropriate amount of protein you should be taking daily. Generally, you should take between 0.6 and 1 gram per pound of lean body mass.

- Let most of your calories from fat come from the good types of fat like the monounsaturated fats, saturated fats, and omega 3s.

- If your net carb limit is low, you should avoid fruits and other low carb treats.

- Don't starve yourself. Ensure that you eat whenever you are hungry. While it helps to keep an eye on your calorie intake, you should never ignore your body needs.

- Drink at least 2-3 liters of water daily.

- Stock up on healthy foods like non-starchy vegetables, meat, eggs, coconut oil, avocado, macadamia nuts, bone broth and other fermented foods, saturated fats, and unsaturated fats.

- Avoid processed fats like vegetable oils, fully and partially hydrogenated oils, margarine, trans fats, soybean oil, corn oil and canola oil.

- Raw and organic dairy products are also good as long as you don't have any allergies. However, you should try to avoid milk due to its high carbs or opt for unpasteurized full-fat milk.

- Increase your electrolyte intake. Ketogenic diets may cause sodium, calcium and potassium deficiency so you should increase intake of mushrooms, salmon and avocados for potassium, nuts or magnesium supplements for magnesium and salt or bone broth for sodium.

- Avoid processed foods as some of the time may contain hidden carbs like sorbitol, maltitol, preservatives, additives and artificial sweeteners. Better still, keep your eyes on the label.

- Ignore any food labeled 'low-fat' or fat-free or low-carb. They would usually contain extra carbs and artificial additives.

- If you are on medications that contain sugars or sweeteners, ask for the sugar-free variety.

- Make sure you always plan your diet in advance to avoid temptations and spontaneous eating.

- Shop weekly and get rid of anything that is not allowed on a diet from your home.

- Have salads and hard-boiled eggs available in case you feel like snacking.

Exercise and the Ketogenic Diet

As we have discussed many times over the course of this book, it is natural to find limitation in your body as soon as you start a Ketogenic diet. But as your body starts adapting to the use of fats as an energy source, you will see that your strength and endurance will soon start coming back to normal.

The question to ask yourself is this: do carbohydrates enable us to build muscle? And the answer to that question is: No, it doesn't. It is still possible to refill the glycogen levels in your body when you are on a Ketogenic diet. The key to that is the amount of protein that you intake.

If that part of the diet is taken care of, you can put on body mass even when you are on a low carb diet. What you can do if you are specifically looking to put on more body weight is that you increase the intake of protein by 1 to 1.2g per lean body mass. It is true that putting on body weight during a Ketogenic diet is slow, but it is only because the total fat content of your body is not increasing as it is getting burnt to provide energy.

People often misquote that Ketogenic diet makes you lose performance. But reports suggest otherwise. A recently concluded test on trained cyclists who were on a low card diet for four weeks showed that they retained the same muscle mass as they had done before they started the diet and there was no dip in aerobic endurance either.

Over the course of the diet, their bodies adapted to the process of using fat as an energy source and limiting both glucose and glycogen stores. Another study conducted on eight gymnasts also seemed to yield the same result.

In the case of both the groups, they were fed green vegetables, proteins, and very high-quality fats. So, this proves that even when you are doing long bouts of cardio, a Ketogenic diet will come across as a hindrance for you.

An exception to this could be an exercise where you are required to an exercise which needs explosive action. To boost your performance during such an exercise you can help yourself to 25-50gms of carbohydrates 30 minutes before starting the training.

You can follow the following steps to know how to exercise when your body is in a state of Ketosis.

Resistance training is a great of way of building muscle as well shed fat, and it does not require you to put in long hours at the gym to do so. You can try lifting in short but intense sessions to fasten the fat burning in your body.

It is advisable to train in shorter sets. The number of repetitions in games should ideally be limited to 10 and repeated numerous times instead of continuing for a long time. The short intervals in between the sets can be utilized by the body to build up any glycogen that it might have lost during the game.

Cardiovascular exercises are ideal applied to perform when the body is in a state of Ketosis.

Although a lot of people will advise against it, eating a small measure of carbohydrates after a workout session enables the sugar contained in the cellulose to travel directly to the muscles.

Fat Loss Plateaus and How to Tackle Them

When you start your diet, you might notice that the extra fat comes off very fast and you lose the weight rapidly and then it gets to some point and you're unable to lose the weight anymore. This is known as a fat loss plateau.

A fat loss plateau on a ketogenic diet may be caused by a number of factors including:

- Eating foods you thought were low in carbohydrates but are actually high in carbs like yoghurt, fruits and nuts.

- Eating a high amount of carbs that spike your insulin levels like artificial sweeteners, sugar alcohols and diary protein.

- Coconut oils are allowed on the ketogenic diet but consuming a lot of it can cause fat loss plateaus. This is because coconut oil contains medium chain triglycerides, which cannot be stored by the body. Your body would have to burn the fat from the coconut oil first and this reduces the amount of stored fat your body burns.

- Lack of exercise is another culprit here. Exercise helps to increase your weight loss results by using up your stored glycogen.

- Excess intake of proteins may also cause fat loss plateaus. An excess of 1.5 kilograms per lean body mass produces the same effect as consuming carbohydrates and could lead to weight gain instead of weight loss.

- Starving yourself by not eating enough food or enough calories would also cause fat loss plateaus because starvation naturally slows down your metabolism and reduces the amount of energy your body burns. On the ketogenic diet, the goal is not to starve yourself but to eat the appropriate foods that would make you stay in nutritional ketosis.

Ending Your Ketogenic Diet the Right Way

You cannot be on a ketogenic diet forever and you definitely shouldn't be. At some point, when you have achieved the results you wanted, you should end your ketogenic diet and start a regular diet that would help you maintain the results you have achieved on the ketogenic diet.

However, many people complain that they found themselves gaining weight after they stopped the ketogenic diet. This is because they didn't end their diet the proper way. So as not to gain back the weight you lose on the diet, there are a few very critical steps you should take.

Introduce carbs slowly: You should avoid over-consumption of carbs when you come off your diet. Instead, you should start introducing carbs slowly at about 20-30 grams daily. Also, to avoid rebound hypoglycemia, you should eat your veggies with starches like rice, pasta and bread.

Control fat intake: After reintroducing carbs into your diet, you should begin to watch your fat intake and make sure it doesn't exceed about 15-20% of your total food intake daily. You can keep your protein consumption stable. However, fat intake shouldn't exceed 50-60 percent of your daily food intake.

Exercise: Exercise is very much needed to maintain the results you would get on the ketogenic diet. After you come off the diet, it is important to ensure that you do not go back to a sedentary lifestyle but do continue to work hard in order to burn the excess calories.

Common Mistakes

- **Intake of Too Many Carbs**

    While this is one of the most common mistakes, this is the cause when you do not do proper research about how much carbohydrates is supposed to be enough according to your body mass index or ideal body weight. A lot of people think that anything under 100 grams per pound is sufficient for you to be able to produce enough ketone bodies to power your body.

    However, as we looked in an example before, with an ideal body weight of 150 pounds, ideally the most about of carbs that you should have is 30 grams only. Only when the carbohydrates are low enough will the body be able to switch from using carbs to power your body to using fats to power your body.

- **Intake of Too Much Protein**

    Protein is one of the most important micronutrient that the body needs to function optimally. Having protein rich food increases fat burning. But, when someone is on a low carb diet, gorging on meat can end up increasing the intake of protein in your body.

    When the body consumes more protein than is required, the protein gets converted into glucose through a process called gluconeogenesis. This glucose gets broken down into sugar that gets used as fuel in your body instead of the fats. It breaks the ketosis state that the body is in.

- **Too Little Intake of Fat**

A human body gets the most amount of calories from the intake of foods rich in carbohydrates. If this source of calories is taken away, then the body will be starved of food to create energy from. Some people, however, think that since having fewer carbohydrates is supposed to be good, so must be the case with having low fats as well.

However, that is one of the biggest myths. Without carbohydrates, the body needs some source of nutrients to use as fuel, and that is when it switches to burn fats into ketone bodies, which does not happen if a number of fats being consumed are also little.

If the carbohydrate and fat, both are taken in lesser quantities, the body will soon run out of energy and starve. As long as you are keeping away from trans-fats and vegetable oils, there is no reason for you to be fearful of fats.

- **Low Sodium Levels**

As soon as the body starts going into a state of ketosis, the insulin levels in the body start going down. One of many uses of insulin is its able to signal the fat cells to store fat. And similarly, the kidney to retain sodium.

When you are on a Ketogenic diet, your body will start losing water, and other minerals including sodium and this are one of the reasons many complain about dizziness, weakness, etc. in the first few weeks of starting a Ketogenic diet. It is because sodium is one of the most important electrolytes that is required by the body for it to function optimally.

The best way to work around this is by taking additional sodium in your food. One of the best sources of food is salt and increasing the intake of salts is one of the best ways of countering this shortage of sodium in the body.

- **Impatience**

Another common mistake, which is very often repeated, is being impatient with the process of ketosis. By default, the body is designed to accept only carbohydrates as a source to fuel the body.

So, if carbs are available to the body, it will always take preference over any other source as a form of energy. When you stop the intake of carbohydrates suddenly, the body needs to get used to burning fats for energy instead of carbs. And it might take a while for the body to burn fat for powering the body primarily. And during this period, as the body gets used to the new source of energy, it is very reasonable for the people undergoing this diet to feel dizzy or sick.

Most people get alarmed as soon as they start feeling under the weather a little bit and resort to discontinuing the schedule and diet as planned earlier. It usually takes anywhere between 2-10 days for the body to adapt to this new mechanism of burning fats completely. It requires you to be patient with yourself and trust the diet that you have planned for yourself.

As I had already mentioned a bit earlier the Ketogenic diet is used by various groups of people for many different reasons. There are medical benefits to following a ketogenic diet such as treatment for diabetes, epilepsy, cancer, heart disease and more. Outside of medical benefits, here are some of the more mainstream and popular reasons why more people are starting to use the Ketogenic Diet:

- **Helps you lose weight fast**

Having a low carb diet is proven to be one of the fastest ways you can go about losing weight. It is even more efficient for weight loss than someone who's on a low-fats diet. This is because a low carbs diet helps to get rid of the excess water from your body, and as your insulin levels lower your kidneys start to shed excess sodium which leads to rapid weight loss.

- **Kills your appetite**

- **Reduces blood sugar and insulin levels**

    When we consume carbohydrates, the food breaks down into simple sugars in our bodies which raise our blood sugar levels. When our blood sugar level rises, our bodies insulin levels rise to minimize the spike in sugar levels to prevent it from harming us.

    Therefore, if you reduce a number of carbs you consume, you can significantly reduce your blood sugar and insulin levels. The Keto diet is a superb solution for diabetics.

- **Blood pressure goes down**

    You can reduce the risk of many common health complications like kidney failures, heart diseases, and many others by decreasing your blood pressure. Consuming fewer carbs is one of the most efficient ways of doing this.

- **Good cholesterol goes up**

    I'm sure we've all heard that high cholesterol can lead to a heart attack, but did you know that there are good and bad cholesterols? The bad cholesterol is known Low-Density Lipoprotein (LDL).

    Too much LDL floating around in your bloodstream is a bad thing which can lead to you having a heart attack. When you reduce the amount of the carbs in your diet, your LDL changes to what's called significant LDL which is benign.

As you can see, there are a lot of upsides to the Keto diet. Unlike many diets you might hear of, the ketogenic diet is not a fad diet. There are many lifelong benefits to it, and it is not as restrictive as you might think. People that follow the Keto diet can still enjoy most foods while maintaining a sober lifestyle.

The Mediterranean-keto fused recipes in this book are crafted so that you get to enjoy great tasting meals while reaping the multitudes of benefits from following a cleaner diet that will transform your body from within.

I hope that you are enjoying this book so far, and if you could spare 30 seconds, I would greatly appreciate you leaving a review on Amazon.com.

Chapter 4

Ketogenic Diet Plan

Metabolically speaking, ketogenic foods are powerful. The surprising benefit is these foods are also delicious, whole natural foods that are extremely healthy for you.

Although there are a number of ways of getting started with a low carbohydrate Ketogenic Diet, most involve a high fat, moderate protein and low carbohydrates plan. What you decide on putting in the plan really hinges on how quickly you want to get yourself into a Ketogenic state.

The more you restrict your body to the intake of carbohydrates, about 15g per day or lower, the faster it is that your body gets into a Ketogenic state. It is advised that the plan contain anywhere between 30g to 60g of carbohydrates for regular dieting. But the lower the amount of glucose in the body, the more desirable the results will be.

A lot of people think that consuming less than 100g of carbohydrates per day is sufficient to take your body to a Ketogenic state but that is not correct. This amount of carbohydrates is too much for a normal human being to achieve Ketosis.

The daily protein requirement should also be monitored and should be just enough as per your body weight. It also depends on how active you are. Too much protein can interfere with the process of Ketosis as well. The remainder of the calories in the meal plan should be in the form of fats. The idea is to get the body into a Ketogenic state and ensure that it stays there.

The intake of nutrients in a diet that is used to induce the body in to Ketosis typically amounts to close to 75% of calories from fats, 20% from proteins and the remaining 5% from carbohydrates. This is when your calories intake is not restricted. A lot of people ask why the protein level is kept moderate and the amount of fats increased. This is because while fats have almost no effect on the blood sugar and insulin levels protein effects both sugar and insulin, if had in large quantities.

If too much protein is consumed than is required as per your body mass, the insulin level in your body rises and this leads to gluconeogenesis which in turn raises the level of glucose in your body. The presence of high insulin and glucose levels in the body can stop the body from burning the fats and producing ketone bodies. A well thought out Ketogenic diet is a powerful tool and hence it is important to understand what it does to your body before you begin.

Before creating a Ketogenic diet for yourself it is imperative that you know the following details about yourself:

1. **Ideal body weight** – this could be the ideal body weight that you should have which can be calculated form multiple websites online or just a weight that you are comfortable being at.

2. Based on the ideal body weight you can also find the total amount of calories that you need to intake to maintain your ideal body weight.

3. Using the guide below, along with your ideal body weight and your daily calorie intake, you can figure out your daily intake of fat, protein and carbohydrates in terms of grams and calories.

Generally, protein intake is supposed to between 1g to 1.5g per kilograms of your ideal body weight. So, if a person has a lean body mass or ideal body weight of 150 pounds or 68 kilograms roughly, the lower limit for his/her protein intake will be 68 grams and the upper limit will be roughly 102 grams. So, the optimal protein intake for such a person will be 68-102 grams per day.

The amount of carbohydrate that you should keep as a part of your daily diet should not exceed 60 grams per day ideally. But that is dependent on how active you are. If you exercise daily, you can consume more food and still in ketosis, but that might come as a challenge for people who are severely resistant to insulin, is diabetic or have other metabolic problems.

Such people may need to further lower their intake of carbohydrates. If your objective to start the Ketogenic diet is weight loss, you should ideally keep the level of carbohydrates below 30 grams per day. If that does not help, you can bring down the intake of proteins to the level of 1g per kilogram of lean body mass or your ideal body weight. If that does not work either, you can reduce the intake of fat as well till your weight starts going down.

The rest of the diet will be made up of fats and oils which can be arrived at by subtracting the calories of proteins and carbohydrates from the total calorie intake. Below is an example of how someone can figure out their intake for number of fat grams.

Say for example that the person under consideration is overweight and wants to come down to an ideal weight of 150 pounds. The daily calorie limit was determined to be 1800 calories per day with 30 grams of carbohydrates and the lower limit of 1 gram per kilogram of body weight. It is important to keep in mind that protein and carbohydrates have about 4 calories per gram of their weight while fats have about 9 calories every gram.

So, the amount of protein which they should ideally intake should be 68 grams or 272 calories (150 pounds is equivalent to 68 kilograms) and the amount of carbohydrates as decided will be 30 grams or 120 calories. This makes it a total of 392 calories of proteins and carbohydrates. What you are left with is 1408 calories of fat that you need to consume per day i.e. about 156 grams of fat.

While there are a number of websites which can give you a direct number instead of having to go through these calculations, most of these numbers that the websites display cannot be trusted as they do not take into account factors such as body, exercise habits and condition of your health. Knowing how to arrive at these numbers is essential so that you can tweak it to your preference.

Examples of Low-Carb Foods

Once you have all the information you need on low-carb foods at your disposal, you can use the following tips to start your diet.

1. The first thing to do would be to head over to your kitchen and remove all high carb foods. This includes any whole grain complex carbs that you might have.

2. The second step should be to replace those stocks by the items mentioned in the lists below.

3. What one needs to understand is that there are no special foods that one needs to purchase to be able to start a Ketogenic diet plan. The only thing that is required is to purchase whole foods that have not gone through too much of processing and are closer to their natural state. The only exception to this rule is artificial sweeteners. Even though they are highly processed, they are better than consuming normal sugar.

4. A Ketogenic diet involves cooking food for yourself, so that you have food which is natural. So be prepared to spend additional hours in the kitchen.

5. It is always advisable to think about what you are going to eat and plan how you to make them beforehand. This is useful so that you buy those things from the grocery store.

6. It is essential that you change your old unhealthy habits and employ new ones in their stead. Instead of going to the usual coffee place and having a cup with bagel, make coffee by yourself at your own home and have it with eggs.

7. If you find yourself getting cramps and headaches when you start the diet, it is possible that you are running low on water in your body. Ensure that you keep yourself hydrated at all time.

Below, you can find the organized lists of all the things that are low on carbs that we need to make a part of our diet. Here is a list of food that have high carbs. You should always avoid these foods at all costs:

- Sugary syrups of any kind, golden syrup, and maple syrup.
- Any kind of brown sugar, demerara sugar, coconut sugar or date sugar
- Caramel
- Corn syrups or sweeteners
- Honey
- Fructose
- Tapioca syrup
- Maltose
- Fruit juice concentrates.

The idea when using sweeteners is to avoid any kind of sugary syrups.

Grain and grain products are also high on carbohydrates and should be avoided, including:

- Breads, rolls or muffins
- Waffles and pancakes
- Pasta
- Cereals
- Tortillas
- Cakes or pies
- Pretzels
- Crackers

You should also keep low on the intake of these foods:

- Any kind of food with corn in it.

- Food with potato in it.

Any other starchy vegetables other than corn and potato like beans, peas, okra and artichokes.

- Canned food products
- Any boxed processed food

Any fruit – most fruits are high on carbs and fructose. Berries have the least amount of carbohydrates among fruits.

Some of the beverages that you might want to avoid are:

- Beers
- Dessert wines
- Sodas
- Milk

All of the food and food products mentioned earlier have either sugar or some form of sugar in them. So, avoiding these foods will help your body sustain ketosis.

Make sure you count all carbohydrates that intake each and every day. Keeping a journal helps in keeping a track of the amount of calories you are taking in every day. Strategize when you are cornered by a social situation. Learn to improvise and stop yourself from eating foods that are high on carbohydrates.

Use the following lists of low-carb foods to help guide you while you prepare your diet:

Fats and oils

☐ Avocado and Avocado Oil
☐ Bacon Fat
☐ Beef Tallow
☐ Butter

- ☐ Chicken Fat
- ☐ Cocoa Butter
- ☐ Coconut Oil
- ☐ Cream Cheese (block)
- ☐ Flaxseed Oil
- ☐ Ghee
- ☐ Heavy Cream
- ☐ Lard (fresh, non-hydrogenated)
- ☐ Macadamia Oil
- ☐ Mayonnaise (full fat)
- ☐ MCT Oil
- ☐ Olives (black or green) and Olive Oil
- ☐ Pork Rinds (fried)
- ☐ Red Palm Oil
- ☐ Salad Dressing (creamy, full fat)
- ☐ Sour Cream (full fat, no fillers)

Sources of Protein

- ☐ Bacon (cooked)
- ☐ Beef (ground, 80-92% lean, cooked)
- ☐ Duck (roasted, with skin)
- ☐ Egg or Egg Whites (whole, large)
- ☐ Lamb (boneless, cooked)
- ☐ Pork Breakfast Sausage (no fillers, no sugar, cooked)
- ☐ Pork Ribs and Pork Shoulder (roasted, plain)
- ☐ Chuck Beef (blade roast, cooked)
- ☐ Beef Steak (broiled or baked)
- ☐ Chicken Breast or Thigh (roasted or baked, no skin)
- ☐ Clams (fresh, baked)
- ☐ Cottage Cheese (1-2%)
- ☐ King Crab (fresh, steamed)
- ☐ Elk Steak (roasted)
- ☐ Flounder, Sole, or Scrod Fish Fillet (no breading, baked)
- ☐ Salmon (fresh fillet or canned pink)
- ☐ Ham (deli style, lean or spiral, smoked)
- ☐ Pork Chops (lean, cooked)

- ☐ Pork Roast Loin (cooked)
- ☐ Scallops (baked or broiled)
- ☐ Shrimp (steamed or boiled)
- ☐ Tuna (canned, water packed)
- ☐ Turkey Breast or Thigh (roasted, no skin)

Vegetables

- ☐ Asparagus (cooked)
- ☐ Beans (black, kidney, chick peas, lentils, cooked)
- ☐ Green Beans (cooked)
- ☐ Blueberries (raw, whole)
- ☐ Broccoli (chopped, cooked)
- ☐ Brussel Sprouts (raw)
- ☐ Green Cabbage (raw, shredded)
- ☐ Baby Carrots (raw)
- ☐ Cauliflower (cooked)
- ☐ Celery (raw, chopped)
- ☐ Cucumber (raw, sliced)
- ☐ Eggplant (raw)
- ☐ Garlic (up to six cloves)
- ☐ Kale (raw, chopped)
- ☐ Lemon or Lime Juice
- ☐ Lettuce (any leaf, shredded)
- ☐ Mushrooms (button or portabella, raw)
- ☐ Onion (white or green, raw)
- ☐ Bell Pepper (raw)
- ☐ Potato (white, cooked)
- ☐ Raspberries (raw, whole)
- ☐ White Rice (cooked)
- ☐ Spinach (raw, cooked, frozen)
- ☐ Spaghetti Squash or Summer Squash (cooked, sliced)
- ☐ Strawberries (raw, whole)
- ☐ Swiss Chard (chopped)
- ☐ Tomato Raw or Tomato Sauce
- ☐ Turnips (raw)

Dairy Products

- ☐ Blue Cheese
- ☐ Brie
- ☐ Natural Cheddar Cheese
- ☐ Cottage Cheese (1-2%)
- ☐ Cream Cheese (block)
- ☐ Mexican Blend Shredded Cheese
- ☐ Monterey Jack Cheese
- ☐ Mozzarella (part skim or whole milk)
- ☐ Parmesan Cheese (hard)
- ☐ Ricotta Cheese (whole milk)
- ☐ Swiss Cheese
- ☐ Heavy Cream
- ☐ Sour Cream (full fat, no fillers)
- ☐ Greek Yogurt (full fat or 0%)

Nuts & Seeds

- ☐ Almond Meal (flour)
- ☐ Coconut Butter
- ☐ Dried Coconut (unsweetened)
- ☐ Almond (roasted)
- ☐ Brazil Nut (roasted)
- ☐ Cashew
- ☐ Hazelnut
- ☐ Macadamia (roasted)
- ☐ Pecan
- ☐ Walnut
- ☐ Peanut (roasted, shelled)
- ☐ Chia Seeds
- ☐ Flax Seeds
- ☐ Pumpkin Seeds (roasted)
- ☐ Sesame Seeds
- ☐ Sunflower Seeds (roasted)

Spices

- ☐ Allspice (ground)
- ☐ Dried Basil
- ☐ Black Pepper
- ☐ Caraway Seed
- ☐ Ground Cardamom
- ☐ Cayenne Pepper
- ☐ Ground Cinnamon
- ☐ Cloves
- ☐ Coriander Seed
- ☐ Ground Cumin
- ☐ Curry Powder
- ☐ Fennel Seed
- ☐ Garlic Powder
- ☐ Ground Ginger
- ☐ Vanilla Extract or Imitation Vanilla Extract
- ☐ Ground Mace
- ☐ Nutmeg
- ☐ Onion Powder
- ☐ Oregano
- ☐ Paprika
- ☐ Dried Parsley
- ☐ Fresh Peppermint
- ☐ Poppy Seeds
- ☐ Poultry Seasoning
- ☐ Pumpkin Pie Spice
- ☐ Ground Sage
- ☐ Dried Spearmint
- ☐ Ground Tarragon
- ☐ Thyme
- ☐ White Pepper

Once again, thank you for reading this book, and I hope you're getting a lot of valuable information. I would greatly appreciate it if you could take 30 seconds to leave me a review for this book on Amazon.com.

Chapter 5

Low-Carb Living Tips for Weight Loss

The low-carb eating in the form of ketosis has a positive effect on hormone regulation-also known as blood sugar regulation, acts a fat burning furnace, and brings the body a number of benefits. Here are seven tips for low-carb living that can help you lose weight...and keep the weight off!

1. Avoid Sugar and Starch

Sugar and starch are a form of carbohydrates, which if consumed in excess, will turn into fat as our liver has no choice to turn that energy into fat and that liver fat leads to further metabolic diseases. Start by limiting your carbohydrate intake to 20 grams a day by avoiding carb-rich foods like flour, pasta, sugar, rice and starchy vegetables. Go through nutrient labels on the consumables and keep a track of your daily carb consumption.

2. Eat "Real Foods"

Medium chain triglycerides (MCT) foods, such as coconut oil, yogurt, and butter consist of good fats, and are easily broken down and used as energy. Highly absorbent, MCTs are commonly used as a therapeutic treatment for malabsorption related issues, including Crohn's Disease. MCTs have also shown benefits when used by people who don't have a gallbladder.

3. Eat Fat to Lose Fat

Although you shouldn't limit yourself to eating meager quantities of oils and butter, you shouldn't consume more once you start feeling full.

4. Eat Greens Every Day

Vegetables are rich with minerals otherwise hard to obtain, like magnesium, potassium, calcium, manganese, folate and betain. The fiber content also speeds up bowel movements, preventing stomach problems while giving the body an overall healthy, refreshing boost. The best way to eat more greens is eating a cup of non-starchy vegetables, raw, and 2 cups of salad greens.

Veggies can include broccoli, summer squash, wax beans, zucchini, jicama, mushrooms, asparagus, Brussels sprouts, leeks, cucumber, eggplant, shallots, rhubarb, celery artichokes, peppers, okra, tomatoes, and pumpkins. It should be remembered that certain vegetables contain a significant amount of carbs, and so should be zigzagged with good fats in your diet.

5. Drink Lots of Liquids

Besides dehydrating yourself with a minimum of 2 liters (at least 8 glasses) of water, drink bouillon to lessen fatigue and headache (unless you are hypertensive). Have a can of caffeinated diet soda or up to 3 cups of coffee a day.

6. Increase Activity While Reducing Stress

Inactive muscles and a stressed mind can go a long way towards impacting the body negatively and making weight loss much harder. Stress may also lead to excessive dietary temptations, like sugar cravings. Increasing the daily activity will keep your mind occupied and manage your sweet tooth while decreasing appetite, building muscle and improving bone density.

7. Eat When You're Hungry, Stop When You're Full

It is great to start off by knowing the difference between hunger and cravings. If you are moderately hungry, feed your body the essential foods so you don't end up wanting more and overeating. If you've had your fair share of food, but are still tempted to eat, distract yourself with activities.

Listen to your body... if you're not hungry you don't have to eat. Even when you eat, make sure you eat until you are not feeling hungry, NOT until you're full. It's better to satiate your hunger 80%, while leaving the 20% intact.

Chapter 6

Tips for Success on the Ketogenic Diet

Just getting started on the ketogenic diet? Good for you! Following are some of the important hacks to remember when following your diet plan in order to get the most out of it, and maximize your success rate.

1. Hydrate Yourself

Your body finds it difficult to retain water when on a ketogenic diet, so replenishing your body with plenty of fluids, especially water is crucial. Drink a minimum of three liters of water a day, and take your urine color as an indicator of proper hydration. A gentle yellow means you are properly hydrated.

2. Remember the Fats

Our bodies need fuel to function. When we restrict our carbs intake, especially to the point where it activates ketosis, back-up fuel is needed by our bodies. Because protein is not a great source of energy, fat is the option our bodies turn to.

The good news is that while in ketosis, most of the fat eaten is turned into energy, and not stored. Therefore, it is important that you choose a wide variety of unsaturated, healthy fat containing foods, like nuts, avocados, dairy products, olives and seeds for consumption.

3. Be Smart About Liqour

Another great perk of the ketosis diet is the ability to enjoy alcohol without compromising your weight loss efforts. Try switching to unsweetened drinks, like scotch, whiskey, vodka, tequila, rum, gin, brandy and cognac while occasionally treating yourself to a low-carb beer.

Low-carb mixers should be your choice of drink, and remember to stay fully hydrated as hangovers are especially bad while in ketosis. Remember to not go crazy as calories still count.

4. Be Patient

Remember that weight loss is not an overnight process, and so don't freak out or lose motivation, and stop weighing yourself every other day! The results are gradual and require persistence and a strong willpower.

Others who are considering purchasing this book would love to know what you think. If you could spare a few seconds, they would greatly appreciate reading an honest review from you. Simply visit the page on Amazon.com.

Chapter 7

Low-Carb Diet Myths Debunked

Before jumping into anything new, we all have questions. If you are curious, and looking for answers regarding the authenticity of myths that soar about low-carb diets, like ketosis, now is the chance to educate yourself. Here we have compiled a list of the 10 most popular myths concerning low-carb diets, and the truth behind these statements.

Myth #1

The low-carb diet is dangerous. The truth is that it is not, and has been proven over the years to be safe and extremely effective. Dr. Atkins gets credit for this diet, but he was not even close to being the innovator, he just brought it into the mainstream, which brings us to myth #2.

Myth #2

William Banting of England who wrote a little booklet titled "Letter on Corpulence Addressed to the Public" is considered the father of low carbohydrate dieting. He proved this over years, helping people lose weight without any side effects.

Myth #3

Low-carbs, high protein and high fat raises cholesterol. The truth behind this statement is it actually lowers cholesterol. For one year, researchers at the Veterans Affairs Medical Center in Philadelphia followed 132 obese adults randomized into two groups.

The carb intake for one group was below 30 grams a day, while for the other, their overall daily caloric intake was reduced by 500 calories with 30% of the calories coming from fat sources. 83% of the study group had diabetes or other risk factors for heart disease.

In the low-carb group, triglyceride levels decreased more and HDL ('good') cholesterol levels decreased less than in the low-fat group. (High levels of triglycerides, a fat in the blood, are associated with heart disease.) People with diabetes on the low-carb diet had better control of blood sugar.

Another research study, published in the Annals of Internal Medicine, involved 120 overweight people and was conducted over a period of six months. Researchers from the Duke University found that participants on the low-carb diet lost 26 pounds, on average, whereas the other group averaged 14 pounds.

The low-carbohydrate group had more beneficial changes in blood triglyceride levels and HDL cholesterol levels than the low-fat diet group. In this study, the low-carb diet groups also received vitamins and other nutritional supplements.

Myth #4

The low carb diet will cause my blood pressure to rise. Again, the truth is with lower LDL levels and VLDL levels, blood pressure levels actually drop. Lead author, Dr. William S. Yancy Jr, associate professor of medicine at Duke, said their findings send an important message to people with high blood pressure who are trying to lose weight.

Myth #5

You need carbohydrates or glucose for your brain to function. The truth is if you are on a hardcore low-carb high protein diet, where carbohydrates are non-existent, you are on what is called a Ketogenic Diet. When on a strict diet, your body produces ketones in the absence of carbohydrates, and then converts the ketones into a form of glucose that enables proper brain function. This brings us to the next myth.

Myth #6

You cannot eat any carbs on a high protein diet. Using the Atkins diet as an example, Atkins himself said on the Larry King show, "You can eat all the carbs your body allows as long as you do not gain weight". What he was talking about was when we reach our desired weight you can add as many carbs to your diet until you start gaining weight, that is your threshold, for some people it is 50 grams a day for others it's 200 grams or more.

Myth #7

I will gain all my weight back if I stop my low carb diet. This is totally false. It does not matter which diet you choose, if you are successful in your weight loss and then stop your diet, 9 out of 10 times you revert back to your old eating habits, and start eating junk and overindulge, then of course you gain weight back.

Myth #8

Eating protein makes you fat. This statement doesn't hold much truth. Protein actually raises your calorie burning metabolism by as much as 30% over carbohydrates. When proteins are consumed, your body must digest and break them down into amino acids. This takes energy and plenty of it, which actually helps you lose weight, not gain it.

Myth #9

High protein diets include fats, and fats are bad for me. Fats in the absence of carbohydrates burn more efficiently, and do not clog your arteries. As the studies show LDL levels (low density lipoproteins) which are the artery cloggers, are lowered. The levels of HDLs, which are the good triglycerides are raised even though your fat intake is increased, that as mentioned above is attributed to low carb intake.

As is previously mentioned, carbs and fat don't mix, and your body cannot efficiently break them down together. Your liver is overburdened and ends up converting the carbohydrates into fat, unless of course you are exercising like crazy.

Myth #10

I will not have any energy with the low carb diet. This statement is totally false, unless you are a marathon runner or bodybuilder. When you consume small amounts of carbohydrates, your body needs another source of energy. When glycogen levels are gone, your body starts using fat for energy and combustion.

If you are extremely active, it will take about 2-3 weeks, after which your body is acclimated to your new eating habits and adjusts, energizing you as before. If you are involved in an endurance sport, then of course you need extra carbs to be competitive. If you are an athlete or workout extensively, you probably would not be dieting anyway, and a low carb high carb is a moot point.

I hope you have learned something from this book so far and would greatly appreciate it if you could leave an honest review on Amazon.com.

Chapter 8

Ketogenic Diet Recipes

Breakfast

1. Keto Pizza Style Waffles

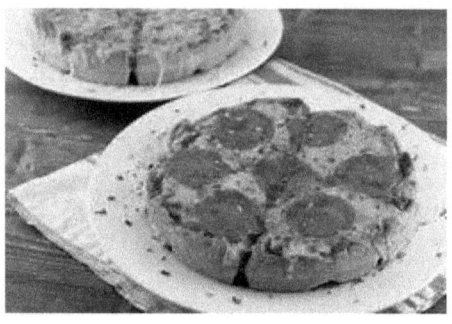

This recipe is perfect for your keto diet and gloriously customizable with your toppings. Let's get started.

Serving size: This recipe will produce two waffles.

Ingredients

- 1 tbsp. butter (or bacon grease)
- One tsp. Baking powder
- 3 tbsp. almond flour
- One tsp. Italian seasoning
- 1 tbsp. psyllium husk powder
- 4 tbsp. parmesan cheese
- 3 oz. cheddar cheese
- Four large eggs
- ½ cup tomato sauce
- 14 pepperoni slices (If you're aiming for a classic pizza)
- Salt and pepper to taste

Directions

1. Add everything except your sauce, cheeses, and toppings to an immersion blender and mix until thick and free of clumps. Heat your waffle iron and add half your blended mixture. Many waffle irons have a handy little light that will tell you when it's ready but if not, look for the flow of steam coming from the iron to almost disappear to indicate it is ready. Repeat step with the rest of your mixture.

2. Add half your tomato sauce (1/4 cup) and half your cheese (1.5 oz.) to each pizza waffle. Add your pepperoni, or any other toppings, to the pizzas.

3. Broil for a few minutes until the cheese begins to bubble and crisp. For cheddar, cooking takes about 3-5 minutes, but this time will vary with other cheese so keep an eye on it! And there you go, two delicious pizza waffles for breakfast. Now go and have a great day!

Nutritional Information (per serving)

Calories: 30
Fat: 2.5g
Carbs: 0.5g
Protein: 1.5g

2. Morning Muffins

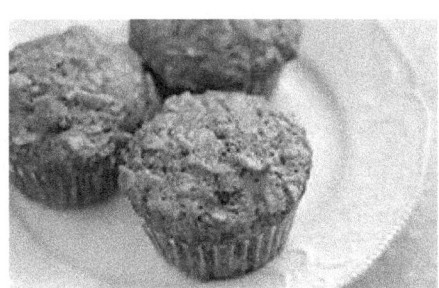

Waking up to a chocolate brownie craving can be such a letdown. You've got your whole day ahead of you but must restrain yourself from the delicious chocolate that's calling your name. No more! This smooth chocolate morning muffin recipe will satisfy your sweet tooth while the addition of pumpkin keeps your keto diet on track.

Serving Size: This recipe will yield six muffins.

Ingredients

- One tsp. Vanilla extract
- 2 tbsp. Coconut oil
- ½ tsp. Salt
- ½ tsp. Baking powder
- 1 tbsp. cinnamon
- ¼ cup cocoa powder
- One tsp. apple cider vinegar
- ¼ cup slivered almonds
- ½ cup pumpkin puree
- One large egg
- 1 cup golden flaxseed meal
- ¼ cup sugar-free caramel syrup

Directions

1. Set your oven to 350F. Combine all your wet ingredients in one bowl and mix well. Do the same to your dry ingredients in a separate bowl. Pour slowly and be sure to mix well to prevent clumping.

2. Set 6 standard paper liners into your muffin tin, and add a roughly ¼ cup of your mixture to each liner. Sprinkle the almond slivers over the tops of the cupcakes for a little garnish and crunch (a dramatic flair while sprinkling is optional).

3. Bake the muffins for 15 minutes, and check. Once the muffins rise and are set, then you'll know they're ready. That's all there is to it! Quick, easy, and your sweet tooth will thank you.

Nutritional Information (per serving)

Calories: 30
Fat: 2.5g
Carbs: 0.5g
Protein: 1.5g

3. Keto Waffles with Pumpkin Spice

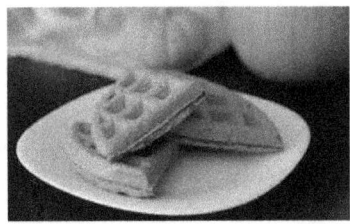

On the keto diet, it's easy to miss our favorite delicious breakfasts. Gazing at a waffle with a sense of longing or grudgingly eyeing someone while they demolish a stack of pancakes is no fun at all. But there is hope for sticking to your diet and enjoying these tasty breakfasts, with the added benefit of pumpkin!

Serving size: This recipe will yield two servings.

Ingredients

- One tsp. baking powder
- One tsp. vanilla extract
- 3 tbsp. swerve sweetener
- 1 ½ tsp. pumpkin pie spice
- 1/3 cup coconut milk
- ½ cup almond flour
- 2 tbsp. flaxseed meal

- ¼ cup canned pumpkin
- Two large eggs
- 7 drops liquid stevia

Directions

1. Mix all your wet ingredients in a large bowl. Be sure to mix well until no egg whites are visible. Combine all dry ingredients in a sifter. If you don't have a sifter, just mixing all the dry ingredients in a bowl and slowly sprinkling them into the wet ingredients will work too. Combine the wet and dry ingredients until they are thoroughly combined. Your mixture will be a little watery, but don't worry!

2. Heat your waffle iron and grease. Coconut spray gives your waffles a vague hint of coconut! Pour your mixture into the iron and cook until the built-in alarm goes off, or the stream of steam begins to dissipate. Serve up with your favorite syrup or fruit!

Nutritional Information (per serving)

Calories: 30
Fat: 2.5g
Carbs: 0.5g
Protein: 1.5g

4. Keto Cheese Tacos

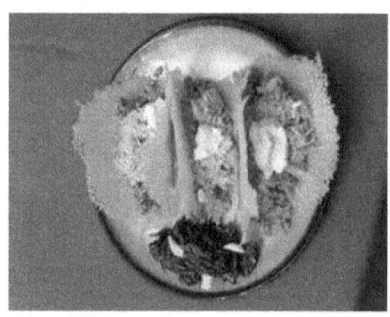

Here we have a refreshing, and quite delectable, take on the traditional taco. Instead of fretting over the flour and carbs used in tortillas, just make your own out of cheese! That's right; eggs, avocado, and bacon wrapped in a crunchy cheese tortilla resulting in the perfect keto friendly start to your day.

Serving size: This recipe will yield three servings.

Ingredients

- Three strips bacon
- 1 oz. cheddar cheese (shredded)
- 1/2 avocado
- 2 tbsp. butter
- 1 cup mozzarella cheese (shredded)
- Six large eggs
- Salt and pepper to taste

Directions

1. Start by thoroughly cooking the bacon. Either in an oven for 15 to 20 minutes at 375F or stovetop. Heat a clean pan over medium heat, and add 1/3 cup of mozzarella. Cook the cheese until it just begins to bubble and turn brown on the side touching the pan. Pay close attention here! Slip a spatula under the cheese and gently unstick it from the pan.

2. Now use a pair of tongs and drape the cheese over a wooden spoon, that should be resting over a bowl or pot. Allow the cheese to cool and form a taco shell shape. Repeat steps with the rest of your mozzarella.

3. Now add your butter and eggs to the pan and cook thoroughly, adding salt and pepper to suit your taste. Divide the eggs equally between your cheese shells. Slice the avocado and divide the slices evenly between the tacos.

4. Chop or crumble your bacon, and again divide equally between the tacos. Last step! Sprinkle your cheddar cheese over the tops. All done!

Nutritional Information (per serving)

Calories: 30
Fat: 2.5g
Carbs: 0.5g
Protein: 1.5g

5. Keto Donuts

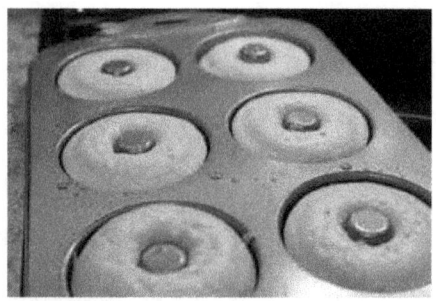

On the keto diet, resisting the pleasure of a staple comfort breakfast food can be a tearful experience. We're of course referring to donuts, but there's hope! Enter the Keto Mini Doughnuts, and those tears of sorrow may flip to joy as you bake these egg, almond, and coconut filled beauties.

Serving size: This recipe yields 22 servings (one donut per serving).

Ingredients

- 4 tbsp. almond flour
- 1 tbsp. coconut flour
- One tsp. vanilla extract
- One tsp. baking powder
- 4 tbsp. erythritol
- 3 oz. cream cheese

- Three large eggs
- 10 drops liquid stevia

Directions

1. Combine with an immersion blender. A food processor will also work for this step if you don't have an immersion blender. Make sure that all your ingredients are well blended and smooth. Heat your donut maker and spray with your grease of choice. Coconut oil always gives your cooking a delicious finish!

2. Pour your mixture into the donut maker. Leave some room (say 10%) to give your donuts space to rise. Let the mixture cook for 3 minutes, and then flip and cook a further 2 minutes. Remove the baked donuts and repeat steps 3 to 5 for the rest of your batter. Voilà! You've just created 22 good keto-friendly donuts.

Nutritional Information (per serving)

Calories: 30
Fat: 2.5g
Carbs: 0.5g
Protein: 1.5g

6. Chive and Bacon Omelet

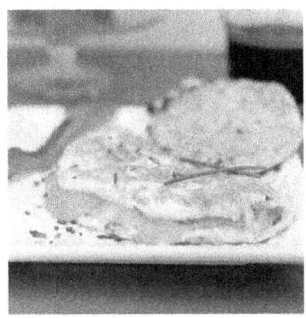

Here we have a simple keto version of the classic bacon and egg omelet. The addition of chive gives this dish a sweet, mellow, onion hint; while the eggs, bacon, and cheese keep this dish firmly in the keto diet's corner. Just a few minutes out of your busy morning and this tasty omelet is all yours!

Serving size: This recipe yields one serving.

Ingredients

- 1 oz. cheddar cheese
- One tsp. Bacon fat
- Two slices bacon (cooked)
- Two stalks cheddar
- Two large eggs
- Salt and pepper to taste

Directions

1. Make sure your chives are chopped, cheese shredded, eggs are cracked and mixed, and bacon cooked before you begin. Omelet making tends to be a fast process so keep on your toes and don't waste time completing these steps later!

2. Heat your bacon fat in a pan on medium-low heat. Add your eggs, chives, and salt and pepper to the pan. Cook until you can see the edges start to set, and then cook for another 30 seconds. Immediately add your bacon to the center of the omelet, and turn off the heat. Sprinkle your cheese on top of the bacon.

3. Fold two edges of the egg on top of the bacon/cheese pile. The melted cheese should hold the egg in place. Repeat step with the rest of the egg. It will create a slightly burrito shaped omelet.

4. Flip the egg over, and allow it to cook a little longer in the pan (it'll still be warm). Feel free to sprinkle some extra chive, cheese, or bacon on top. There you go! A very fast paced recipe, but it'll leave you with a delicious start to the day.

Nutritional Information (per serving)

Calories: 460
Fat: 36g
Carbs: 2g
Protein: 25g

7. Brie and Raspberry Stuffed Waffles

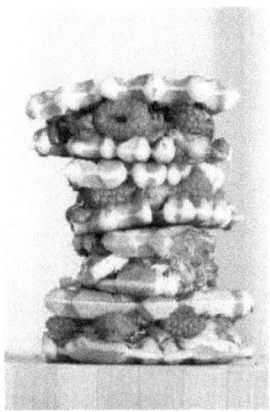

Start your day with panache and elegance as you whip up this unique creation. To call it a simple breakfast sandwich would be to offer insult, and here's why! This little gem takes almond flour and coconut milk to create keto friendly waffles; then fills them with a zesty combination of raspberry and brie to create a morning meal that will have you strutting out your door ready to take on the world.

Serving size: This recipe yields two servings.

Ingredients for the Waffles

- One tsp. vanilla extract
- One tsp. baking powder
- 2 tbsp. flaxseed meal
- 1/2 cup almond flour
- 2 tbsp. swerve sweetener

- 7 drops liquid stevia
- Two large eggs
- 1/3 cup coconut milk

Ingredients for the Filling

- 1 tbsp. lemon juice
- 1 tbsp. swerve sweetener
- 2 tbsp. butter
- 3 oz. cream brie

Directions

1. Mix all the waffle ingredients in a container. Make sure your batter is smooth with no lumps. Heat your waffle maker, and once it's hot, add your mixture. Cook until either the indicator light says its ready or the steam dissipates. Remove your waffles and repeat as necessary to cook all of your batters.

2. Slice your brie and drape over two of your four waffles. The waffles will still be warm, and this will melt the brie. In a pan, heat the swerve sweetener and butter. Just as the butter begins to bubble; add your raspberries, lemon juice, and zest. Stir your raspberry mixture until it starts to boil. As the mixture lets off steam, it will develop a jam-like consistency, and this is what you want!

3. Now take the two waffle pieces with the brie, and broil them until the brie begins to bubble. Pour/spread your raspberry jam on top of the brie waffles and cover with the other two waffles. Grill the assembled waffle sandwich in the pan for a couple of minutes until brown and crispy. Enjoy!

Nutritional information (per serving)

Calories: 490
Fat: 40g

Carbs: 6g
Protein: 22g

8. Baked Avocados with Eggs and Bacon

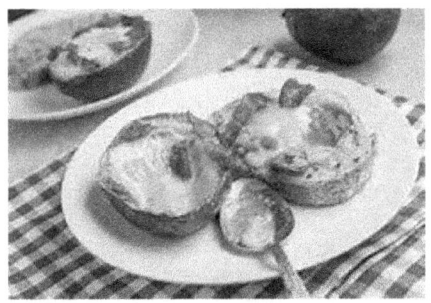

We've all heard of stuffed peppers for dinner, but how about stuffed avocados for breakfast! Easy to make, and using just avocado, bacon, eggs, and pepper, these cups of early morning goodness are yours for the taking!

Serving size: This recipe yields one serving.

Ingredients

- Two small eggs
- Two slices of bacon
- 1 avocado
- Pepper to taste

Directions

1. Pan fry your bacon until it is just barely cooked. Preheat your oven to 425F. Halve the avocado and remove the seed. Crumple some aluminum foil into ring shapes that will hold your avocado halves up on the baking sheet. Break your eggs into a bowl, and spoon one yolk into each avocado half. Then continue to fill the hole of each avocado with egg whites until they're both full.

2. Crumble your bacon, and spread on top of the avocados. Add pepper on top, and bake in the preheated oven for 12 to 15 minutes. After 10 minutes, check your eggs every minute or two to ensure you don't overcook them! Serve them up!

Nutritional information

Calories: 700
Fat: 60g
Carbs: 6g
Protein: 23g

9. Greenie Protein Smoothie

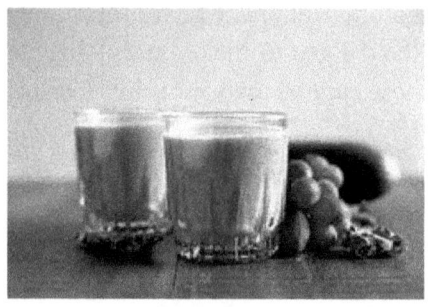

Sitting down to a pleasant, hot, morning breakfast is certainly a fantastic start to the day; but whether it is work, school, or only being trapped under those comfortable blankets until the last moment, those rushed mornings always appear. However; you can be ready with this quick breakfast smoothie that saves on carbs while packing on the healthy fats to keep your diet running strong.

Serving size: This recipe yields one serving.

Ingredients

- One scoop/0.9 oz. vanilla (or plain) whey protein powder (egg white powder)
- 2 tbsp. pistachio nuts

- One tsp. vanilla extract
- 6 drops liquid stevia
- 1/4 cup fresh spinach
- 1/4 cup coconut milk
- 1/4 cup fresh mint
- 1/2 avocado
- 1/2 cup water
- Ice cubes (if desired)

Directions

1. Rinse your mint and spinach. Peel and halve the avocado, and remove the seed. Add all ingredients to a blender or food processor, and blend until smooth. All done! Easy, right?

Nutritional Information (per serving)

Calories: 490
Fat: 37g
Carbs: 9.5g
Protein: 26g

10. Lavender Biscuits

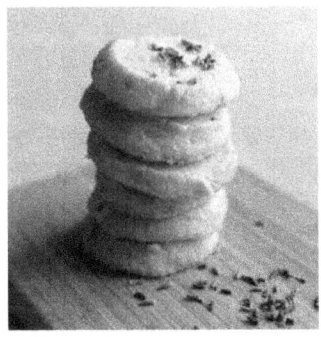

Wake up feeling classy and ready for a suitably suave breakfast? Then look no further than these low carb purple biscuits. Easy to make, packed with almond flour, and to boast a subtle lavender finish; these cookies are perfect for a light and tasty breakfast. To take your game to the next level, check out our recipe for low carb peach jam as the perfect sidekick to these biscuits!

Serving size: The recipe makes six servings.

Ingredients

- Four eggs whites
- 1/3 cup coconut oil
- 1 1/2 cups almond flour
- 1 tbsp. lavender buds (culinary grade)
- One tsp. baking powder
- 4 drops liquid stevia
- One pinch kosher salt

Directions

1. Combine the coconut oil and almond flour in a bowl. Your hands would be the best tool for this job, and mix until there are pea-sized clumps of fat throughout the mixture. Put the bowl of flour and oil in the refrigerator.

2. Whip your egg whites until they begin to foam, and add the salt, lavender, and baking powder. Mix well. Add oil, and mix well. Use a tablespoon or ice cream scoop to place clumps of the mixture on a greased baking sheet. Give each mound a slight pat, so they're not round (think puffy pancake). Bake at 350F for 20 minutes or until golden brown. Enjoy!

Nutritional information (per serving)

Calories: 270
Fat: 25g
Carbs: 4g
Protein: 10g

11. Peach Chia Jam

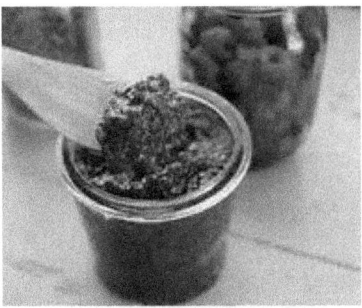

Chia seeds have the very useful tendency to form a jelly-like consistency when mixed with liquid; which makes them the perfect choice for whipping up smoothies, jams, and puddings without using commercial gelatins. Here we'll call on these little fellows to help us put together a delicious jam consisting of peaches, chia seeds, low-carb sweetener, and lemon.

Serving size: This recipe yields ten servings.

Ingredients

- 2 tbsp. swerve sweetener
- 2 tbsp. chia seeds
- One tsp. Lemon juice
- 2 cups peaches (chopped)

Directions

1. Combine your peaches, lemon juice, and sweetener in a blender; and blend until completely smooth. Pour the smooth mixture into a bowl and add your chia seeds. Stir by hand until completely incorporated. Pour your jam mixture into a jar or covered bowl, and place in the refrigerator. All done! Quick recipe and this jam will be the perfect accompaniment for many of your favorite breakfast pastries!

Nutritional information (per serving)

Calories: 30
Fat: 1g
Carbs: 3g
Protein: 1g

12. Keto Style McMuffin

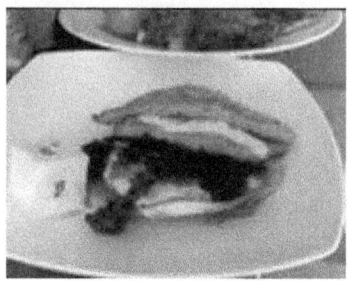

Who would have thought that you could enjoy a fast food breakfast sandwich while on the keto diet? But guess what? You can! The Keto Style McMuffin combines all the tastiness of its namesake but slashes the carbs and ups the healthiness.

Serving size: The recipe yields two servings.

Ingredients for the Muffins

- One large egg
- tbsp. heavy whipping cream
- 1/4 tsp. baking soda
- 2 tbsp. water
- 1/4 cup cheddar cheese (grated)
- 1/4 cup flax meal
- 1/4 cup almond flour
- One pinch salt

Ingredients for the Filling

- Two slices cheddar cheese
- One tbsp. butter
- 1 tbsp. ghee
- Two large eggs
- 1 tsp. dijon mustard
- Four slices crisp bacon
- Salt and pepper to taste

Directions

1. Add all your dry ingredients for the muffins in a large bowl and mix well. Drop in the eggs, cream, and water. Mix until completely smooth. Add the grated cheese to the mixture and stir again. Don't worry if the cheese makes it clumpy when you heat it everything will combine nicely. Add your mixture to two single serving ramekins, and microwave on high for 60 to 90 seconds.

2. For the filling, cook your eggs on top of the ghee. Don't worry if they're not perfect circles. Do your best, and you can trim later.

3. Now cut the cooked muffins in half, and spread your butter on each half. Now stack up! Layer your egg, mustard, bacon, and cheese for each muffin. Enjoy! All the deliciousness of the classic McMuffin but completely guilt free!

Nutritional Information (per serving)

Calories: 315
Fat: 55g
Carbs: 3g
Protein: 26g

13. Goat Cheese and Spinach Omelet

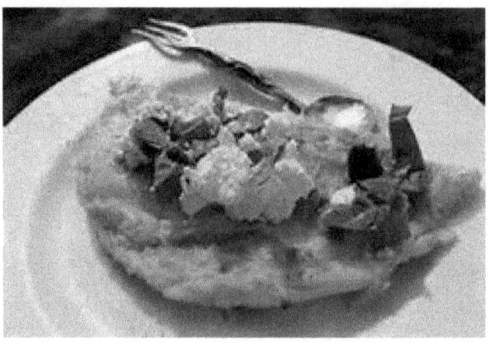

Omelets are the reliable go-to breakfast for the keto diet. The eggs and cheese are bursting with healthy fats and protein, while you can still tailor each one to your tastes with an endless array of fillings. This goat cheese and spinach option is one such combination; we hope you enjoy!

Serving size: The recipe yields one serving.

Ingredients

- Three large eggs
- One medium spring onion
- One large handful of spinach
- 2 tbsp. heavy cream
- 2 tbsp. butter
- 1/4 onion
- 1 oz. goat cheese
- Salt and pepper to taste

Directions

1. Spread the butter on the pan until it is completely melted. Slice your onion (or dice it), and add to the pan once the butter begins to brown. Caramelize your onion in the butter. Once the onion is fully cooked and caramelized, add your spinach to the pan. Cook until the spinach is wilted. Add salt and pepper to taste, give a

final stir, and remove the spinach onion mix from the pan and set aside.

2. Now crack your eggs in a container (not the pan!), and add the cream and some salt and pepper. Mix everything together. Now you can add your egg mixture to the pan, and cook until the edges just begin to set.

3. Add your onion spinach mixture on one side of the egg, covering about half of the eggs. Crumble your goat cheese over the onion and spinach. Fold the other half of the egg over top of the onions, spinach, and cheese. Remove from pan and garnish with more cheese if you like (who doesn't like more cheese?). Serve it up and enjoy!

Nutritional information (per serving)

Calories: 615
Fat: 58g
Carbs: 5.4g
Protein: 26g

14. Creamy Coconut Yogurt

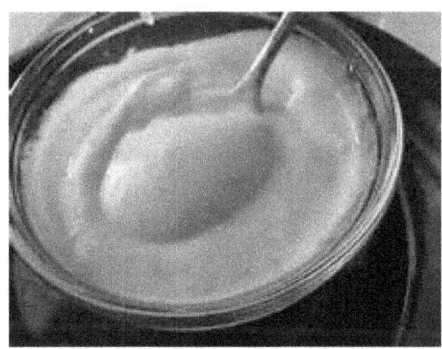

Wake up with a hankering for something savory, creamy, and delicious; but feel too guilty to have pudding for breakfast? Then grab this recipe for Creamy Coconut Yogurt! Coconut milk, cream and any toppings you like to give your day a scrumptious start!

Serving size: This recipe yields about 2.5 cups of yogurt, and 1/2 cup equals one serving.

Ingredients

- 2/3 cup heavy whipping cream
- Two capsules probiotic-10
- 1/2 tsp. xanthan gum
- One can use coconut milk (full fat)
- toppings (your choice!)

Directions

1. Pour the contents of your can of coconut milk into a container and stir well as the water and cream tend to separate (you can do this directly in the can too). Put your coconut milk in a sealable container, and break the probiotic capsules into the milk, mix well, seal the container, and place in the oven (with the heat off and the oven light on). After the sitting time, add your yogurt to a bowl and sprinkle in your xanthan gum. Mix altogether.

2. In a separate bowl, use an electric mixer to whip your fat milk until stiff peaks form. Add the cream to the yogurt, and mix until you get the consistency you want. Add whatever toppings you wish. Any berry is sure to be delicious! Enjoy your own, homemade, yogurt!

Nutritional Information (per serving)

Calories: 310
Fat: 31g
Carbs: 4.5g
Protein: 0.5g

15. Keto Pumpkin Donut Holes (with cardamom)

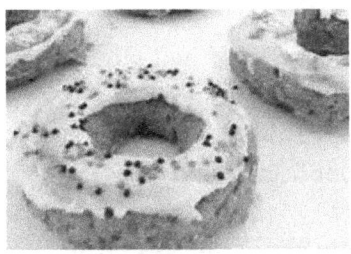

Donut holes for breakfast? On the keto diet? Oh yes indeed, we've got you covered. These donut holes will keep you on your diet, and the addition of cardamom and pumpkin give these beauties a wonderfully unique taste.

Serving size: The recipe yields 12 servings/donut holes.

Ingredients

- 1/4 tsp. vanilla extract
- 1/4 tsp. salt
- 1/4 tsp. orange extract
- One tsp. cardamom
- 3/4 tsp. liquid stevia
- 2 tbsp. erythritol
- 1 cup pumpkin puree (100%)
- 1/3 cup butter (melted)
- 1/2 cup coconut flour
- Three large eggs

Directions

1. Melt your butter in the microwave. Add your eggs, vanilla extract, orange extract, and stevia to a large bowl. Mix well. In a separate bowl, combine your flour, erythritol, cardamom, and salt. Now combine your egg mixture, pumpkin, and butter. Mix until smooth. Sift, or slowly add, the dry ingredients into the wet,

stirring as you go. You should have a sticky, dough-like, mixture by now.

2. Roll the dough into golf ball sized balls and place them in a cupcake tray. Bake at 325F for 18 to 25 minutes, or until they begin to brown. Dust with cinnamon or any sweetener if you wish. Wow, your friends and enjoy!

Nutritional Information (per serving)

Calories: 92
Fat: 7.5g
Carbs: 2.5g
Protein: 2g

16. Keto Style French Toast Muffins

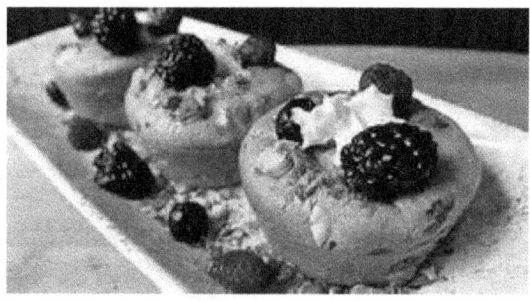

Everyone loves muffins. Everyone loves French toast too. So why not combine them? Or better yet, why not combine them AND keep them on the keto diet. Well, friends, we've done just that.

Serving size: The recipe yields 11 servings/muffins.

Ingredients

- One tsp. cinnamon
- 2 tbsp. erythritol
- 1 tsp. vanilla extract

- 1 tbsp. butter (unsalted)
- 2 tbsp. coconut oil
- 1/2 tsp. salt
- 1/4 tsp. nutmeg
- 1/4 cup heavy cream
- 1/4 cup peanut butter
- 1/4 cup toasted almonds (crushed)
- Six large eggs
- 2/3 cup almond flour
- 10 drops liquid stevia

Direction

1. Preheat your oven to 350F. If your almonds aren't already toasted, grind them up in a food processor and add them to a pan heated to medium-high. Keep a close eye on them and stir occasionally. Add your peanut butter, coconut oil, and butter to a bowl and microwave until completely melted (about 40 seconds). Mix completely.

2. Combine your erythritol, salt, cinnamon, almond flour, and nutmeg in a separate bowl. Combine your melted butter mixture, the dry ingredients, and the heavy cream. Stir and mix completely. Divide the mixture evenly in a cupcake tray and top with your toasted almonds. Bake for approximately 20 to 25 minutes.

3. Give them about 5 minutes after removing from the oven to cool, and then remove from the cupcake tray. Allow them to cool for at least 15 minutes and top with whipped cream. Serve them with a sprinkling of extra cinnamon or some berries if your wish!

Nutritional Information (per serving)

Calories: 170
Fat: 16.5g

Carbs: 2.5g
Protein: 7g

17. Flax Seed and Almond Pancakes

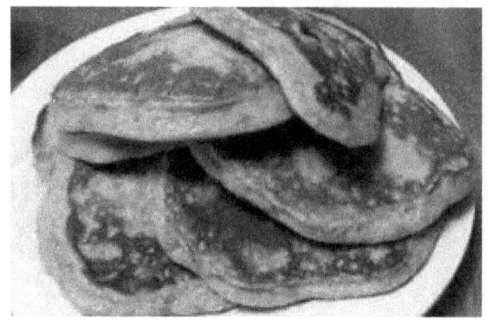

Ah yes, pancakes! Stacks and stacks of pancakes practically awash in syrup. You don't have to give up on these dreams with the keto diet. Our pancakes using almond flour and flax seeds keeps the carb count down will stacking the odds for fats and protein.

Serving size: The recipe yields eight pancakes/servings.

Ingredients

- Four large eggs
- 2 tbsp. erythritol
- One tsp. Baking powder
- 1/2 tsp. nutmeg
- 2 tbsp. butter
- 1 tbsp. coconut flour
- 1/2 tsp. cinnamon
- 4 tbsp. coconut oil
- 1/2 cup almond flour
- 1/2 cup flax seed meal
- 1/2 cup coconut milk
- Pinch of salt

Directions

1. Combine all the ingredients. Mix all your wet ingredients (except butter and coconut oil) in a separate bowl. Make sure ingredients are well combined and smooth. Add the wet ingredients to the dry, constantly stir to get a smooth consistency. Heat your pancake pan/griddle on medium-high, and grease with butter and coconut oil.

2. Add approximately 1/4 cup of your mixture to the pan. Once bubbles form on top, allow to them to cook for another 30 seconds and then flip. Repeat for the rest of your mixture. Serve them up! Some sugar-free or homemade syrup would be the perfect accompaniment.

Nutritional information (per serving)

Calories: 215
Fat: 19g
Carbs: 2g
Protein: 6g

18. Waffle Disguised as Cinnamon Roll

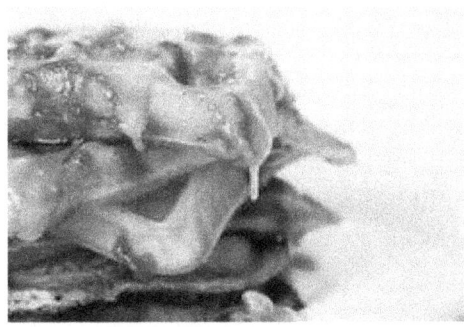

Just as we offered you French toast combined with muffins, we suggest a similarity sweet (in both senses of the word) combination to get your morning rolling, waffles and cinnamon rolls! Our low carb takes on these two favorites will keep you on the keto diet while providing a mouth-watering breakfast that your friends will covet.

Serving size: The recipe yields one serving.

Ingredients for the Waffle

- 1/2 tsp. cinnamon
- 1/2 tsp. vanilla extract
- 1/4 tsp. baking soda
- Two large eggs
- 1 tbsp. erythritol
- 6 tbsp. almond flour

Ingredients for the Frosting

- 1/4 tsp. vanilla extract
- 1 tbsp. erythritol
- 1/4 cinnamon
- 1 tbsp. heavy cream
- Two tsp. batter from waffles
- 2 tbsp. cream cheese

Directions

1. For the waffles, mix all dry ingredients in a bowl. In a separate bowl, mix all your wet ingredients together. Ensure that everything is mixed thoroughly. Add the wet ingredients to the dry, mix until smooth. Heat your waffle iron. When hot, add your batter and begin cooking. Remember to reserve two tsp. for the frosting.

2. While the waffle is cooking, add your cream cheese and erythritol to a small bowl. Now add the cinnamon, heavy cream, and butter. Mix completely, so the mixture is smooth. Once the waffle is

finished cooking, remove from the iron, and spread your frosting over the top. Serve and enjoy!

Nutritional Information (per serving)

Calories: 545
Fat: 52g
Carbs: 6g
Protein: 25g

19. Deviled Eggs with Bacon

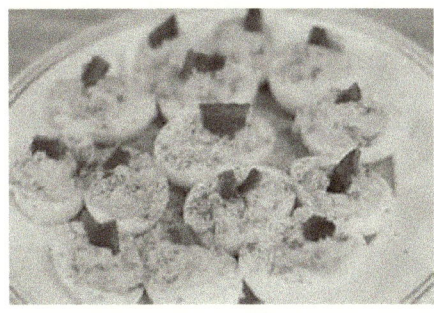

Deviled eggs aren't just a fancy appetizer! Whip up these little devils with some bacon and a smidge of cayenne pepper to create a wonderfully satisfying and zippy breakfast for yourself.

Serving size: The recipe yields three servings.

Ingredients

- One tsp. dijon mustard
- 1/2 tsp. rosemary
- 1 tbsp. bacon fat
- 1/4 tsp. cayenne pepper
- Two slices bacon
- 1/4 cup mayonnaise (preferably homemade)
- Five large eggs (hard boiled)

Directions

1. Slice/chop your bacon and toss them into a pan on medium heat. Remember they will shrink a little as they cook so don't cut too small! Slowly cook the bacon until it is fully cooked and crispy. Cut your hard-boiled eggs in half, and scoop out the yolks.

2. Add the eggs, mayo, cayenne pepper, bacon fat, mustard, and half of your rosemary to a bowl and mix. Add some of your crispy bacon to the holes left by the removed yolks, and fill the rest of the way with your egg mixture. Now garnish with the rest of your bacon and the remaining rosemary. Enjoy!

Nutritional Information (per serving)

Calories: 330
Fat: 29g
Carbs: 2g
Protein: 15g

20. Sausage Frittata

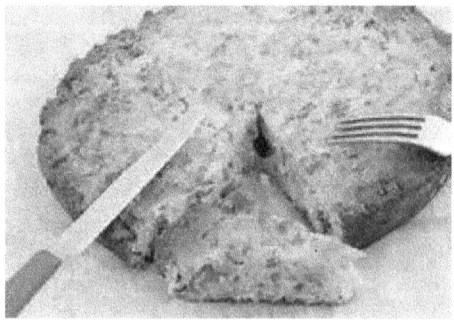

Big day ahead? Fill up with this keto hearty egg frittata stuffed with sausage to get your engine revved and ready for your day.

Serving size: The recipe yields 20 slices/servings.

Ingredients

- 3/4 cup onion
- 2 cups cheddar cheese
- One medium green pepper
- 7 cups spinach
- 1/2 lb. Italian sausage
- 1/2 lb. chorizo
- 12 large eggs
- 8 tbsp. heavy cream
- 1 tbsp. olive oil
- One tsp. Garlic powder

Directions

1. Fry the olive oil add the spinach. Once the spinach wilts and cooks down, remove from the pan and start cooking the chorizo and sausage. While this cook, crack the eggs into a large bowl, add the heavy cream, and all spices. Mix altogether.

2. Preheat your oven to 350F. When the sausage is cooked and crumbled, add it to the same reserve bowl as the spinach, but keep the sausage fat in the pan. Now add your chopped onion and some pepper to the pan, and cooking until translucent. Add to bowl with spinach and sausage when done.

3. Now add your egg mixture to all your cooked ingredients and mix thoroughly. Put the whole mixture in a foiled, and buttered pan. Bake for approximately 45 minutes or when you can run a knife through the frittata, and it comes up clean. Slice it up and serve!

Nutritional Information (per serving)

Calories: 175
Fat: 14g
Carbs: 1.2g

Protein: 12g

21. Scrambled Eggs with Spinach and Cheddar

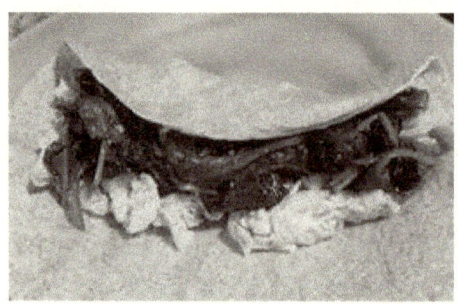

Classic scrambled eggs are the perfect breakfast for the keto diet. Lots of fats and protein and this recipe takes scrambled eggs to the next level by adding cheese and some spinach.

Serving size: The recipe yields one serving.

Ingredients

- 1 tbsp. olive oil
- 1 tbsp. heavy cream
- 1 pinch each of salt and pepper
- Four large eggs
- 4 cups spinach
- 1/2 cup cheddar cheese

Directions

1. Add the heavy cream, salt, and pepper TO THE EGGS. Mix to your desired consistency. Heat a large pan and throw in your olive oil. When hot, add the spinach and as it begins to sizzle and wilt, add a little salt and pepper.

2. When the spinach is fully cooked and wilted and reduce heat to medium and add the egg mixture. Stir slowly as the eggs begin to

cook. When the eggs have set, dump your cheese on top and allow to melt. Enjoy!

Nutritional Information (per serving)

Calories: 700
Fat: 55g
Carbs: 7g
Protein: 42g

22. Sausage and Feta Omelet

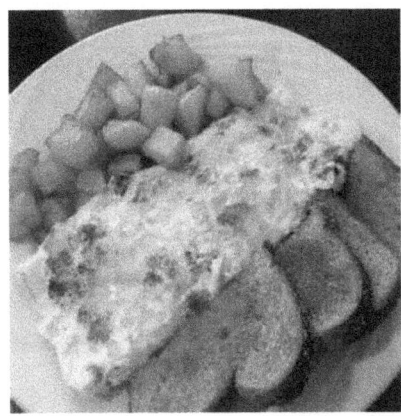

A filling omelet bursting with sausage and feta cheese is just the thing to start your day! Easy to make, this egg will help keep your hunger, and diet, in check!

Serving size: This recipe yields one serving.

Ingredients

- 1/2 tbsp. olive oil
- 1/4 cup half and half
- 1 tbsp. feta cheese
- Two sausage links
- Three large eggs

- 1 cup spinach
- 1 pinch black pepper and salt.

Directions

1. Heat two pans on medium, and add your oil to one of them. Mix your eggs with the half and half in a bowl, and add all your seasoning to this egg mixture. Toss your sausage links into the pan that does not have the oil. Add spinach to the pan with the oil. Monitor the two pans, and when everything is cooked put it all in a single large bowl. Add your egg mixture to the pan with the sausage fat.

2. When the edges of the eggs begin to set, add the sausage, spinach, and cheese. Give it one more minute to cook, then flip half of the egg over to cover the insides. Flip the whole omelet, and cook for a further 2 minutes. It helps if your cover the pan and allow the steam to cook the eggs as well. Enjoy!

Nutritional Information (per serving)

Calories: 540
Fat: 42g
Carbs: 2.5g
Protein: 30g

23. Classic Bacon and Eggs

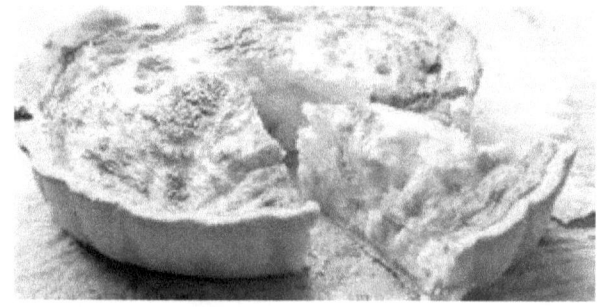

No breakfast recipe list is complete without the classic bacon and eggs. Follow our simple recipe and enjoy this comforting meal.

Serving size: This recipe yields one serving.

Ingredients

- 1 tbsp. butter
- 1 pinch each of salt and pepper
- Three large eggs (room temperature)
- Four slices bacon
- 1/3 cup heavy cream

Directions

1. Preheat your oven to 350F. Place the bacon on an oven sheet, and cook for 15 minutes until crispy. Whisk your eggs and cream. Be gentle as you whisk, we're not trying to beat the eggs.

2. Heat a pan on medium-low, and add the butter. Once the butter has melted, add your egg mixture. Let sit until the eggs begin to set, then begin to stir. Remove from the pan when the eggs are still ever so slightly runny, add your bacon, salt, and pepper. Enjoy!

Nutritional Information (per serving)

Calories: 695
Fat: 65g
Carbs: 2.5g
Protein: 28g

24. Keto Pumpkin Pancakes

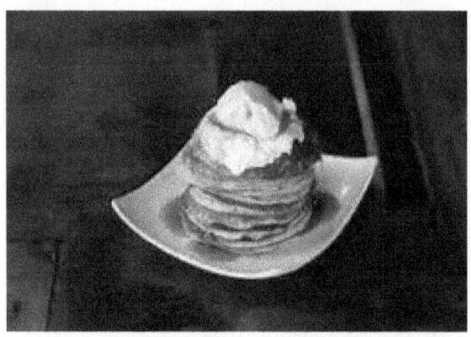

Well, let's not leave pumpkin pancakes out! This keto friendly recipe will let your whip up some truly delicious pancakes that are still great at any time of the year!

Serving size: The recipe yields eight servings.

Ingredients

- One tsp. pumpkin pie spice
- 2 tbsp. butter
- 1 tsp. baking powder
- 1/4 tsp. salt
- 1/4 cup pumpkin puree
- 1 cup almond meal
- 1/4 cup sour cream
- Two large eggs

Directions

1. Combine your sour cream, butter, and eggs. In a separate bowl, mix the baking powder, spice, salt, and almond meal. Now slowly add the wet ingredients to the dry while stirring continuously. It Will give you a nice smooth batter. Heat a cast iron skillet on medium, and grease with butter. Pour about 1/3 cup of your batter onto the skillet.

2. When bubbles begin to form on top, let cook for another minute, and then flip. Cook for one more minute. Repeat steps for the rest of your batter. Serve up with your favorite toppings!

Nutritional Information (per serving)

Calories: 150
Fat: 11g
Carbs: 1.5g
Protein: 5.5g

25. Keto Quiche

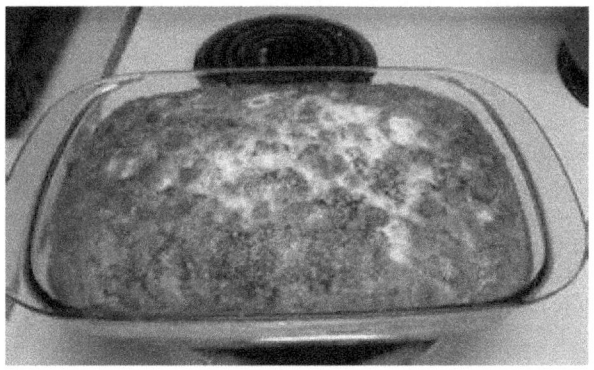

Have guests for breakfast? Then impress them with this delicious, keto friendly, quiche recipe. Or whip it up on the weekend and keep it all to yourself!

Serving size: This recipe yields eight slices/servings.

Ingredients for the Crust

- 1/4 cup olive oil
- 1/4 tsp. salt
- 1 tsp. oregano (dried)
- 1 1/2 almond flour

Ingredients for the Filling

- 1/2 tsp. pepper
- 1/4 tsp. salt
- 1 tsp. garlic
- 1 tsp. Mrs. Dash (table blend)
- 1 1/2 cups cheddar cheese
- One green bell pepper
- Six large eggs
- Six slices of bacon

Directions

1. Preheat your oven to 350F. Slice your bacon into good sized chunks, and add them to a stovetop pan heated on medium. Add ALL of the crust ingredients to a bowl and use your hands to mix. When fully mixed, form a ball and press the dough into an 11x7 casserole dish. It won't be cooked all the way! It will continue to cook as the fillings bake.

2. When the bacon finishes cooking, remove and add the green peppers and garlic to the pan. Cook in the bacon fat while keeping the pan on medium heat.

3. In a separate bowl, combine all the seasoning, cheese, eggs, bacon, pepper, and garlic. You can toss in the fat from the pan if you wish. Pour the mixture into the crust and bake for 16 to 18 minutes. Allow to cook and enjoy!

Nutritional information (per serving)

Calories: 330
Fat: 30g
Carbs: 3.8g
Protein: 11.5g

26. Keto Chicken Frittata

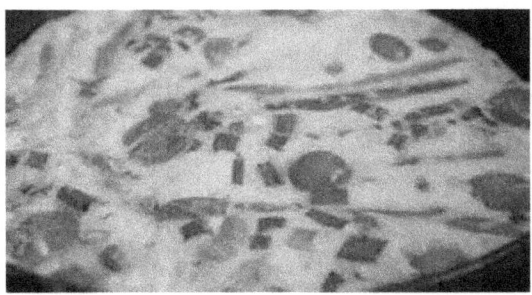

This chicken frittata is for you! Healthy chicken baked into an egg pie; this keto recipe is overflowing with healthy fats and protein.

Serving size: The recipe yields eight slices/servings.

Ingredients

- 1 1/2 cup cheddar cheese
- Ten large eggs
- 2 1/2 Bella mushrooms (chopped)
- 3 cups spinach (chopped)
- Three chicken sausages
- 2 tsp. hot sauce (your choice)
- 1 tbsp. ranch dressing
- 1/2 tsp. Mrs. Dash (table blend)

Directions

1. Preheat oven to 400F. Chop your sausages, and start cooking in a cast iron skillet on medium high. We're aiming for nice and crisp sausages here. When the sausages are approaching cooked, toss in the spinach and mushrooms.

2. In a separate container, crack the eggs and mix with your ranch, hot sauce, and spaces. Mix everything completely. Once the spinach and mushrooms are cooked, pour in your eggs as well as

the cheese. Give this several stirs to make sure everything is combined in the pan. Now slide your pan into the oven for 10 minutes. Finish it up with a 3 to 4-minute broil. Slice it up and serve!

Nutritional information (per slice)

Calories: 235
Fat: 18g
Carbs: 3g
Protein: 20g

27. Keto Breakfast Layer

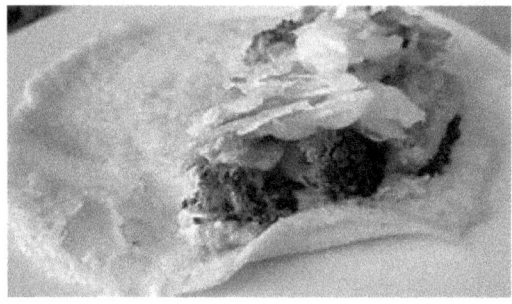

Feeling utterly ravenous? It cooks up this breakfast made of layers of bacon, egg, and cheese! Perfect for getting your cheese and bacon craving under control.

Serving size: This recipe yields four servings.

Ingredients

- 1/4 tsp. salt
- 1/4 tsp black pepper
- 2 tbsp. heavy cream
- 1/4 tsp. Mrs. Dash (table blend)
- 4 cups spinach
- Four large eggs

- Ten slices bacon
- 2 tbsp. bacon grease
- 1/2 cup cheddar cheese

Directions

1. Preheat oven to 400F. Weave your bacon into about a 5x5 slap. Think of how a basket weave works, but with bacon! Bake the bacon weave for about 25 minutes, until fully cooked. Remove and place on paper towel. Add your bacon grease to a stovetop pan, and toss in the spinach.

2. Add the eggs and all the seasoning. Slowly scramble the eggs until thoroughly cooked. Spread the cooked eggs on top of the bacon weave. Beat the eggs with the cheese and broil for 4 minutes. There you go! Let it cool and then cut into four pieces.

Nutritional Information (per serving)

Calories: 305
Fat: 26g
Carbs: 2g
Protein: 18g

28. Keto Coffee Cake

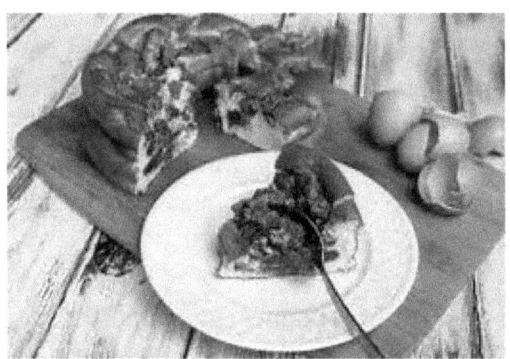

Coffee cake isn't just for the carb carefree anymore! Follow this recipe in using almond flour for your cake, and you'll get to enjoy this delicious breakfast indulgence too!

Serving size: This recipe yields eight slices/servings.

Ingredients for the Base

- 1/4 tsp. liquid stevia
- 1/4 tsp. cream of tartar
- Two tsp. Vanilla extract
- 1/4 cup protein powder (unflavored)
- Six oz. cream cheese
- 1/4 cup erythritol
- 6 eggs (separated)

Ingredients for the Filling

- 1/2 stick butter
- 1/4 cup erythritol
- 1 tbsp. cinnamon
- 1 1/2 cup almond flour
- 1/4 cup maple syrup substitute

Directions

1. Preheat oven to 325F. Add your egg yolks and erythritol to a bowl, and cream. Add all remaining ingredients for the base (except cream of tartar and egg whites), and whisk together. Slowly fold 1/2 of the egg white mixture into the egg yolks mixture. Be gentle as you complete this process! Now add the remaining 1/2.

2. Now, in a separate container, mix all of the ingredients for the filling. Mix until a dough forms. Pour your base mixture into a metal cake pan. Top with half of the sauce. You may have to push

this down a little if it doesn't sink through on its own. Bake for 20 minutes, and then add the rest of the filling to the top. Bake a further 25 to 30 minutes. A toothpick inserted in the middle should come up clean. Let cool for 20 minutes and then remove. Enjoy!

Nutritional Information (per slice)

Calories: 255
Fat: 25g
Carbs: 3.2g
Protein: 13g

29. Keto Chive Soufflé

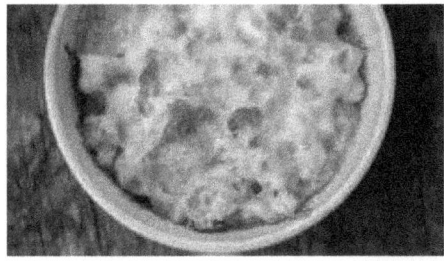

This delicious soufflé combine cheese, ham, and eggs will start your day on the right path. Stuffed full of healthy fats as well to keep you on the keto diet!

Serving size: The recipe yields five servings.

Ingredients

- 1 tbsp. butter
- 3 tbsp. fresh chives (chopped)
- Six large eggs
- 6 oz. ham steak (cooked and cubed)
- 1 1/2 garlic (minced)
- 1/2 onion (diced)

- 3 tbsp. olive oil
- 1 cup cheddar cheese
- 1/2 cup heavy cream
- 1/2 tsp. salt
- 1/4 tsp. black pepper

Directions

1. Preheat oven to 400F. Heat olive oil in a stovetop pan. Once hot, add your onions. Continue to cook until they begin to brown.

2. In a separate bowl, mix the rest of the ingredients. Once combined, add the onion and garlic to the mix. Divide the mixture evenly between 5 ramekins. Bake for approximately 20 minutes. Allow to cool and enjoy!

Nutritional Information (per serving)

Calories: 400
Fat: 41g
Carbs: 3g
Protein: 20g

30. Breakfast Burger with Peanut Butter

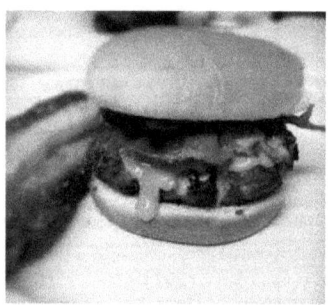

Burger for breakfast? We've got you covered. But we're changing things up with the addition of peanut butter!

Serving size: This recipe yields 2 servings.

Ingredients

- Two large eggs
- 1 tbsp. butter
- Four slices bacon
- 1 tbsp. PB fit powder
- 2 oz. pepper jack cheese
- 4 oz. sausage
- Salt and pepper to taste

Directions

1. Preheat oven to 400F. Bake your bacon in the oven for 25 minutes, or until thoroughly cooked. Mix the butter and PB fit powder together. Set this aside for later use. Use your hands to form the sausage into the traditional burger patty shape. There should be 2.

2. Cook these patties on a stovetop pan over medium heat. Once cooked, add the cheese and cover with a pan to allow it to melt. Now separately cook your eggs over easy. Assemble! Arrange the burger, eggs, and bacon to make your breakfast burger stack, and top with the PB butter mixture. Enjoy!

Nutritional Information (per serving)

Calories: 650
Fat: 55g
Carbs: 3.5g
Protein: 29g

31. Breakfast Keto Pizza

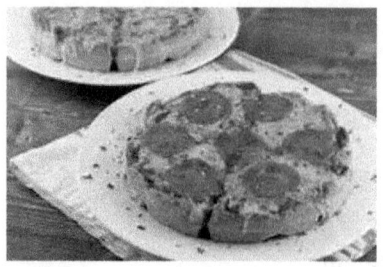

Serving size: This recipe yields 2 servings.

Ingredients

- Ten slices of Pepperoni
- 4 Eggs
- 2 ounces of Cheddar Cheese
- 4 slices of Bacon
- Onion Powder
- Garlic Powder
- Pepper
- Salt

Directions

1. Cook your bacon and reserve your bacon grease in your skillet. Let your pan cool off for a bit. Crack your eggs into your pan and put them all close together. Apply your seasoning. Cook at 450 degrees in your oven for approximately 6 minutes. Add your toppings and cheddar. Cook for about four more minutes. Place your bacon on top. Serve!

Nutritional Value

307 Calories.
22 grams of Protein.
1 gram of Carbs.
24 grams of Fat.

32. Breakfast Meatloaf

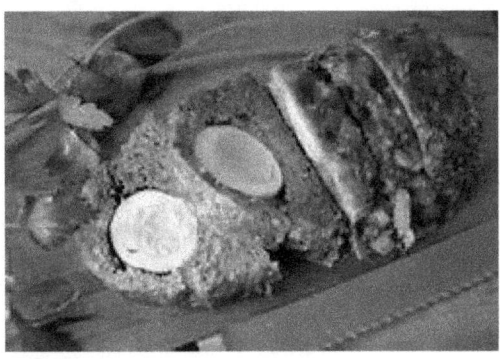

Serving size: This recipe yields 4 servings.

Ingredients

- 6 Large Eggs
- 4 ounces of Organic Cream Cheese (Room Temperature)
- 1 pound of Sweet Italian Sausage or Breakfast Sausage
- 1 cup of Shredded Cheddar Cheese
- 1/4 Yellow Onion (Chopped)
- Two tablespoons of Chopped Scallion
- Ghee

Directions

1. Preheat your oven to 350 degrees. Grease your small-sized loaf pan with your ghee. In your large-sized bowl, lightly beat your eggs. Add your sausage, onion, and half of your cream cheese. Mix thoroughly. Pour your meatloaf and egg mixture into your loaf pan. Add to your oven and bake, uncovered, for approximately 30 minutes or until stiff.

2. Remove from your oven and allow it to sit for about 5 minutes. Some of your fat may have risen to the top and begun to cool. You can use your spoon to scrape it off lightly. Spread your remaining

cream cheese over the top of your meatloaf, then top it with your scallions and cheddar cheese. Add your meatloaf back to the oven. Broil for about 2 to 3 minutes or until your cheddar cheese begins to golden and crisp. Remove from your oven. Allow your meatloaf to rest for at least 5 minutes before slicing. Serve!

Nutritional Value

682 Calories.
38 grams of Protein.
5 grams of Carbs.
56 grams of Fat.

33. Keto Cinnamon Crunchy Granola

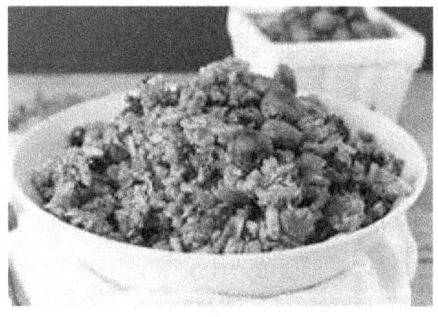

Serving size: This recipe yields 4 servings.

Ingredients

- 1 cup of Sliced Almonds
- 1 cup of Diced Walnuts
- Oil 4 packs of Splenda Naturals
- Two teaspoons of Cinnamon

Directions

1. Preheat your oven to 375 degrees. Line your baking sheet with your parchment paper. In your medium-sized bowl, toss all your

ingredients together. Spread out your mixture over your baking sheet in as close to a single layer as you can.

2. Add to your oven and bake for approximately 10 minutes, or until your mixture begins to brown. Remove, mix again and place in your bowl with some cold unsweetened almond milk. Serve!

Nutritional Value

562 Calories.
14 grams of Protein.
16 grams of Carbs.
54 grams of Fat.

34. Keto Cacao Nibs Cereal

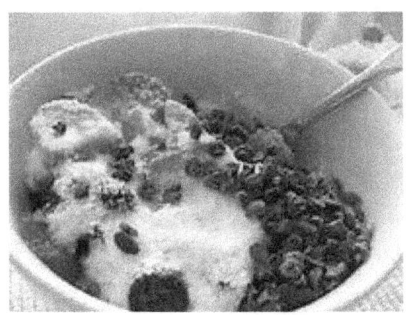

Serving size: This recipe yields 4 servings.

Ingredients

- Two tablespoons of Raw Cacao Nibs
- 1/2 cup of Chia Seeds
- Four tablespoons of Hemp Hearts
- Two Tablespoons of Melted Coconut Oil
- One tablespoon of Fine Psyllium Powder
- 1 tablespoon of Organic Vanilla Extract
- 1 cup of Water

- 1 tablespoon of Swerve

Directions

1. Preheat your oven to 285 degrees. In your large-sized mixing bowl, combine your chia seeds and water, stir well and allow it to sit for approximately 5 minutes. Add the rest of your ingredients to your bowl, except for the cacao nibs.

2. With your electric mixer or wooden spoon, mix all your ingredients together well until they are evenly amalgamated. Add your cacao nibs and stir them into your dough. The dough should form a nice ball of pliable consistency.

3. Roll out two large-sized pieces of oven paper, about 11x14-inches. Take your dough and using your hands form it into a cylinder. Place it on your parchment paper with the shiny side up.

4. With your fingers start flattening the dough. Cover it with the other piece of your paper, shiny side down, and roll it out with a rolling pin to a thickness of 1/4 to 1/8-inch. Gently peel off the top paper from your dough. Lay your dough on top of the paper on your cookie sheet or the top part of your broiler pan.

5. Bake on one side for approximately 15 minutes or until almost dry. Remove from your oven and carefully flip your sheet of dough. It should be dry enough to take off your oven paper, peeling it gently.

6. Bake for another 15 to 25 minutes or until dry. Remove from your oven and allow it to cool. Using a large kitchen knife cut your cereal into 1-inch squares. Serve!

Nutritional Value

254 Calories.
9 grams of Protein.

1.5 grams of Carbs.
15.5 grams of Fat.

35. Keto Scrambled Eggs

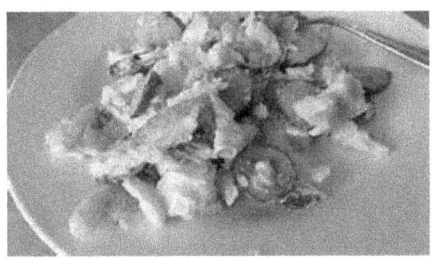

Serving size: This recipe yields 2 servings.

Ingredients

- 6 Eggs
- Four strips of Bacon
- Two tablespoons of Sour Cream
- 1/2 teaspoon of Onion Powder
- 1/2 teaspoon of Garlic Powder
- 2 tablespoons of Butter
- 1/4 teaspoon of Paprika
- 1/4 teaspoon of Black Pepper
- 1/2 teaspoon of Salt
- Green Onion (Optional)

Directions

1. Crack your eggs into your ungreased, cold pan and then add your butter. Wait to mix your eggs until you put the heat on. Don't season your eggs until after they are cooked. It will break them down and make them watery instead of creamy.

2. Put your pan on medium-high heat. Start stirring your butter and eggs together using your silicone spatula. While stirring your

eggs, cook some bacon strips in a different pan to your desired level of crispiness.

3. Alternate stirring your eggs both on heat and off the heat. A few seconds on and a few seconds off the flame. If the eggs begin cooking in a thin, dry looking layer at the bottom of your pan, take if off heat. Scrape it using your spatula and that thin layer should regain some of its creaminess.

4. Once your eggs are almost done turn off the flame. Your eggs will still cook a little more due to the residual heat in your pan. Add two tablespoons of your sour cream. Season your eggs using your pepper, salt, garlic powder, paprika, and onion powder. Add in a couple of stalks of chopped green onion for some different flavor if you so desire. Serve!

Nutritional Value

444 Calories.
25 grams of Protein.
2 grams of Carbs.
35 grams of Fat.

36. Deep Fried Eggs

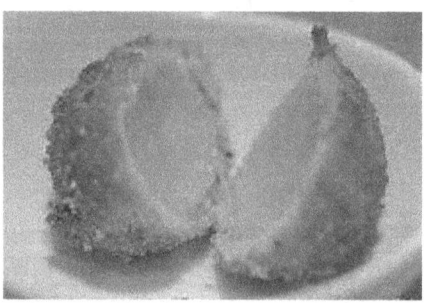

Serving size: This recipe yields 1 serving.

Ingredients

- Three slices of Bacon
- 2 Eggs

Directions

1. Fry the oil. Cook your bacon. Crack your eggs into your prep bowl. Slip your egg into the center of your fryer. Don't drop eggs in, try to slip your eggs in near the surface.

2. Using two different spatulas, corral your eggs into a ball. It may take a little practice to get the hang of. Fry for approximately 3 to 4 minutes or until the bubbling stops. Drain on your paper towels. Serve!

Nutritional Value

321 Calories.
27 grams of Protein.
1 gram of Carbs.
24 grams of Fat.

37. One Skillet Eggs & Bacon

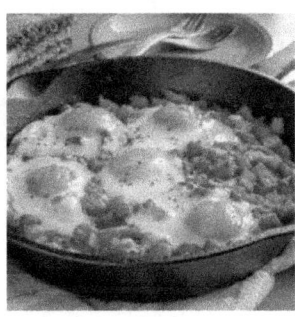

Ingredients

- 4 Large Eggs

- 1/2 cup of Shredded Colby Jack Cheese
- Eight slices of Bacon
- 1/2 cup of Chopped Cauliflower or Broccoli
- 1 tablespoon of Butter
- 1/2 Cup of Finely Chopped Celery
- 1/2 Large Chopped White Onion.
- 1 Peeled Carrot

Directions

1. Slice your bacon across its grain into smaller-sized strips. Melt your butter in your large-sized skillet over medium heat. Add your bacon and vegetables. Stir often and saute your vegetables and bacon in your butter for approximately 20 minutes. You want your bacon to begin crisping on its edges, and you want your plants to being caramelizing.

2. Spread your mixture over your skillet as evenly as possible and make four wells one in each quarter of your skillet. Break an egg into each of the wells. Cook your eggs until they are nearly done. Cook shorter if you like your yolks runny and longer if you like them harder. When your eggs are nearly done sprinkle cheese on top and allow it to cook until your cheese melts, and the eggs are done. Serve!

38. Ricotta Scrambled Eggs

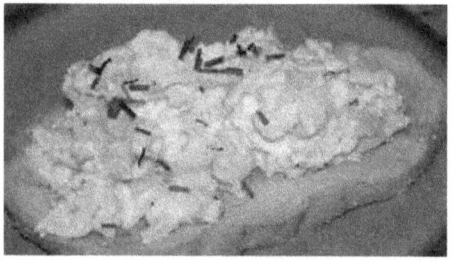

Serving size: This recipe yields 1 serving.

Ingredients

- 2 Eggs
- 2 ounces of Italian Dry Salami
- 5 ounces of 2% Fat Ricotta Cheese
- 1 tablespoon of Olive Oil
- One teaspoon of Rosemary
- Salt
- Pepper

Directions

1. Chop your salami up into smaller-sized cubes. Fry them together in your small-sized pan using olive oil. While frying, whisk your eggs, add your salt, pepper, and rosemary. Add your ricotta into your egg mixture, mix well to break up any large-sized lumps. Add your eggs and ricotta mixture to your pan and cook for approximately 5 minutes until done. Serve!

Nutritional Value

598 Calories.
28 grams of Protein.
5 grams of Carbs.
45 grams of Fat.

39. Keto Sausage & Egg Muffin

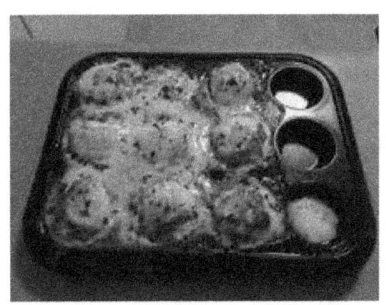

Serving size: This recipe yields 1 serving.

Ingredients for the Muffin

- 1 Egg
- One tablespoon Coconut Flour
- One tablespoon Almond Milk
- One pinch of Salt

Ingredients for the Filling

- 1 Sausage Link
- 1 slice of Cheese
- 1 Egg
- 1/4 teaspoon of Sage
- 1/4 teaspoon of Thyme
- 1/8 teaspoon of Black Pepper
- 1/4 teaspoon of Salt

Directions

1. Preheat your oven to 400 degrees. Crack your egg into your mixing bowl and add each of your muffin ingredients. Mix well. Get rid of any clumps and pour your batter into your ramekin. Bake for approximately 15 minutes. Crack your egg into your ramekin. Give your egg a good stir and season with your salt and pepper. Bake for about 10 minutes. Cut open your pork sausage link and discard its casing.

2. Add your seasonings to your sausage meat and mix using your hands. Shape them into a patty and then cook using your hot pan for approximately 4 to 5 minutes on both sides. Remove from the oven and cut your muffins into thin halves. Toast them until they are browned. Put together your sandwich and add your slice of cheese. Serve!

Nutritional Value

460 Calories.
29 grams of Protein.
3 grams of Carbs.
37 grams of Fat.

40. Cali Chicken Omelet

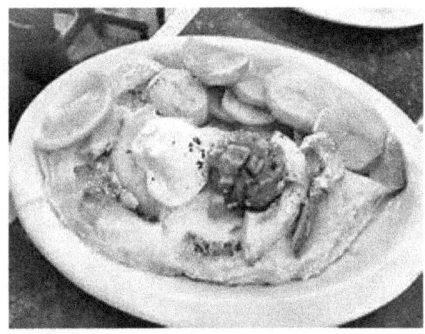

Serving size: This recipe yields 1 serving.

Ingredients

- 1 ounce of Deli Cut Chicken
- 2 Eggs
- 1 Campari Tomato
- Two slices of Bacon (Chopped & Cooked)
- One tablespoon of Mayo
- 1/4 Avocado
- 1 teaspoon of Mustard

Directions

1. Crack your eggs and beat them in your small-sized bowl. Add to your hot pan. Pull sides of your eggs towards the center to cook your omelet faster. Season them with your pepper and salt.

2. Once your eggs are half cooked, should take approximately 5 minutes, add your bacon, tomato, chicken, and sliced avocado. Add in your mayo and mustard. Fold your omelet over onto itself. Cover using your lid. Cook until finished. Should take approximately 5 minutes. Serve!

Nutritional Value

415 Calories.
25 grams of Protein.
4 grams of Carbs.
32 grams of Fat.

41. Breakfast Lettuce Taco

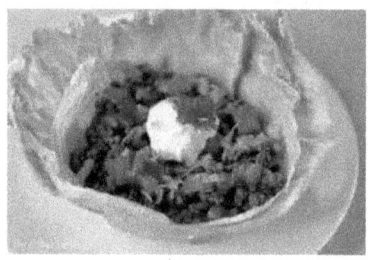

Serving size: This recipe yields 2 servings.

Ingredients

- 4 Large Eggs
- Six slices of Bacon
- 2 slices of Cheddar Cheese
- 2 tablespoons of Heavy Cream
- 2 tablespoons of Shredded Cheddar
- 2 Romaine Lettuce Leaf
- Onion Powder
- Pepper
- Salt

Directions

1. Cook your bacon to your desired preference. Whisk your eggs, cream, and add your seasonings.

2. Scramble your eggs and mix in your cheese at the end. Combine your eggs, cheese, bacon, and lettuce. Serve!

Nutritional Value

499 Calories.
29 grams of Protein.
3 grams of Carbs.
40 grams of Fat.

Lunch

42. Berry & Chicken Summer Salad

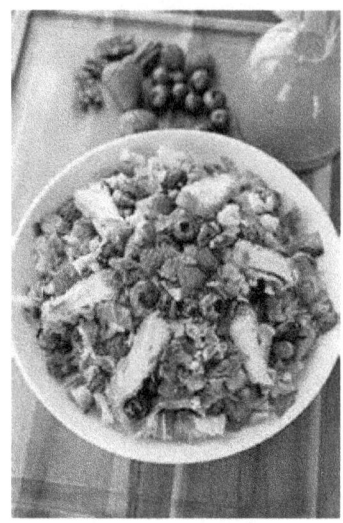

Serving size: This recipe yields 2 servings.

Ingredients

- 1 Chicken Breast
- 3/4 cup of Blueberries
- 6 Diced Strawberries
- Three tablespoons of Raspberry Balsamic Vinegar
- 2 cups of Spinach
- 1/2 cup of Chopped Walnuts
- 3 tablespoons of Crumbled Feta Cheese

Directions

1. Cut your chicken breast up into small-sized cubes and cook in your pan.

2. Gather your other ingredients and add them to your large-sized bowl. Add your dressing. Add your chicken and toss your salad. Serve!

Nutritional Value

335 Calories.
21 grams of Protein.
16 grams of Carbs.
19 grams of Fat.

43. Grilled Halloumi Salad

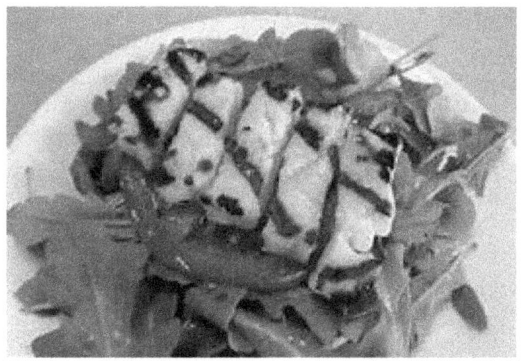

Serving size: This recipe yields 1 serving.

Ingredients

- 5 Grape Tomatoes
- 1 Persian Cucumber
- 1/2 ounce of Chopped Walnuts
- 3 ounces of Halloumi Cheese
- Handful of Baby Arugula
- Olive Oil
- Balsamic Vinegar
- Salt

Directions

1. Cut your halloumi cheese into approximately 1/3-inch sized slices. Grill your slices for approximately 3 to 5 minutes on both sides. Should have nice grill marks on each side. Prep your salad by washing then cutting your vegetables. Cut your tomatoes in half and cut your cucumbers into smaller slices. Chop your walnuts and add them in your salad bowl.

2. Wash your baby arugula and add to your bowl. Arrange your grilled halloumi cheese on top of your salad. Add some salt. Dress your salad with your balsamic vinegar and olive oil. Serve!

Nutritional Value

560 Calories.
21 grams of Protein.
7 grams of Carbs.
47 grams of Fat.

44. Keto Mini Chicken Pot Pies

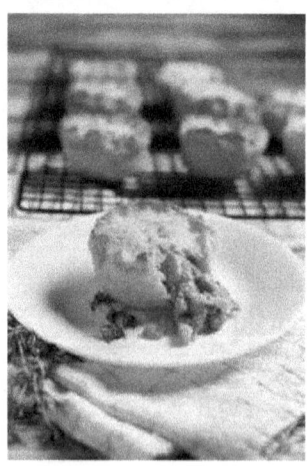

Serving size: This recipe yields 12 servings.

Ingredients for the Filling

- 1 pound of Diced Chicken Breast
- 1 Medium Diced Onion
- Two tablespoons of Butter
- 1/2 cup of Coarsely Grated Carrot
- 2 stalks of Finely Chopped Celery
- One tablespoon of White Wine Vinegar
- 1/4 teaspoon of Dried Thyme Leaves
- 1 1/2 cups of Heavy Cream
- 1/2 cup of Chicken Stock
- Two teaspoons of Paprika
- Pepper

Ingredients for the Crust

- 2 Large Eggs
- 1 cup of Almond Flour
- 1/2 cup of Coconut Flour
- Ten tablespoons of Butter
- Two teaspoons of Baking Powder
- 3 cups of Part-Skim Mozzarella Cheese (Grated)
- 1/4 teaspoon of Dried Thyme
- 1/4 teaspoon of Sea Salt

Directions

1. Begin by preparing your filling. Over a medium-high heat melt one tablespoon of butter in your large-sized skillet. When your butter stops foaming add your diced chicken. Brown, your chicken on all sides, then sprinkle lightly with your salt and pepper. Remove your chicken to a plate and set to the side for later.

2. Heat your same skillet to medium and add one tablespoon of butter. When your butter has stopped foaming add your onions,

dried thyme, celery, and to your skillet. Cook, frequently stirring until your onions are slightly brown on the edges and cooked through.

3. Add your white wine vinegar and stir, scraping up any browned bits. When your vinegar becomes syrupy add the broth. Turn the heat to high until your soup simmers, then turn to low and simmer broth and vegetables until broth is reduced and slightly thickened.

4. Stir in your cream and paprika. Simmer on low until thickened. Add your chicken, peas, and any drippings into the sauce and briefly reheat. Sprinkle to taste with your salt and pepper. Turn off your heat and set to the side until your crust is ready to fill.

5. Add your almond flour, coconut flour, baking powder, salt and, dried thyme to your medium-sized mixing bowl. Mix thoroughly using your whisk. Break eggs into your small-sized bowl. Whisk to break up your yolks. Add your eggs to your dry ingredients and stir. A silicone scraper works well for this process. The mixture will be mealy.

6. Place your large-sized saucepan over a low heat. Add your butter and mozzarella cheese. Stir constantly until your butter and cheese are melted. Do not be concerned if they remain separated. When both your cheese and butter are melted, remove from the heat and add your flour and egg mix, stirring rapidly. They do not have to combine thoroughly.

7. Pour your mixture out onto one of the pieces of parchment paper. While your dough is hot (but not hot enough to burn hands), knead it to mix in your flour mixture thoroughly. Working quickly, cut your larger section of dough into 12 equal sections. Roll each section between 2 pieces of parchment paper to about a four 1/2-inch circle. Press each circle into your cup on your muffin tin.

8. Spread Out the remaining third of your dough. Spoon your filling evenly into the bottom crust in the muffin cups. Do not over-fill. If you have extra filling, serve it with the pot pies to pour over the top.

9. Top each of your mini pot pies with a circle and pinch the edges to seal. Place your muffin tin on your cookie sheet. Bake your pot pies in your preheated oven for about 17 to 22 minutes or until the tops are a golden brown. 5 minutes before removing them from your muffin pan.

Serve!

Nutritional Value

445 Calories.
23 grams of Protein.
6 grams of Carbs.
36 grams of Fat.

45. Keto Kale & Sausage Soup

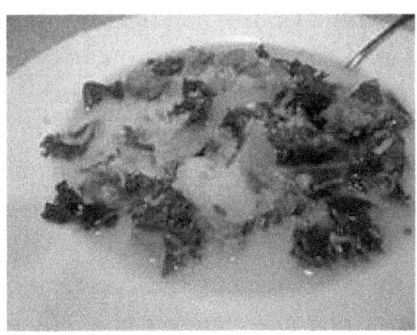

Serving size: This recipe yields 6 servings.

Ingredients

- 1 pound of Sweet Italian Sausage (Ground)

- 1 Medium Carrot (Peeled & Diced)
- 1 Medium Yellow Onion (Chopped)
- One tablespoon of Butter
- Two cloves of Crushed Garlic
- 1 teaspoon of Dried Oregano
- Two tablespoons of Red Wine Vinegar
- 1 teaspoon of Dried Rubbed Sage
- One teaspoon of Dried Basil
- 4 cups of Low-Sodium Chicken Broth
- 3 cups of Chopped Kale
- One teaspoon of Sea Salt
- 1/2 teaspoon of Freshly Ground Black Pepper

Directions

1. Heat your large-sized saucepan or Dutch oven over medium-high heat. Add your ground sausage, breaking up your meat. Cook, until browned and cooked through. Should take approximately 5 minutes. Using your slotted spoon, remove your cooked sausage and allow to drain on a plate covered with your paper towels. Discard the drippings, but do not wash your pan. Melt your butter over medium heat. When the bubbling subsides, add your onion and carrot. Cook until your onion begins to brown on the edges and becomes somewhat translucent.

2. Stir your garlic into your onion and carrot mixture. Cook for approximately 1 minute. Add your red wine vinegar and cook until syrupy, scraping up any browned bits. Should take about 1 minute. Stir in your oregano, basil, sage and red pepper flakes. Pour in your stock and heavy cream. Increase the heat to a medium high.

3. When your soup reaches a simmer, add your cauliflower and turn the heat down to a medium-low. Simmer uncovered until your cauliflower is fork-tender. Should take about 10 minutes. Stir in your kale and cooked sausage. Cook 1 to 2 minutes longer, or

until your kale wilts and your sausage is reheated. Season with your salt and pepper. Serve!

Nutritional Value

298 Calories.
16 grams of Protein.
6 grams of Carbs.
24 grams of Fat.

46. Apple & Ham Flatbread

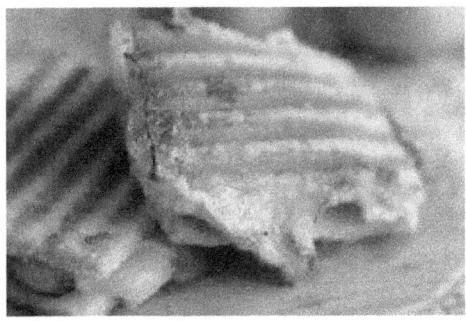

Serving size: This recipe yields 8 servings.

Ingredients for the Crust

- Two tablespoons of Cream Cheese
- 3/4 cup of Almond Flour
- 1/8 teaspoon of Dried Thyme
- 1/2 teaspoon of Sea Salt
- Ingredients for the Topping:
- 1 cup of Mexican Cheese (Grated)
- 4 ounces of Low Carbohydrate Sliced Ham (Cut into Chunks)
- 1/4 Medium Apple (Seeded, Cored, & Unpeeled)
- 1/2 Small Red Onion (Cut into Thin Slices)
- 1/8 teaspoon of Dried Thyme
- Salt

- Pepper

Directions

1. Preheat your oven to 425 degrees. Cut two pieces of parchment paper about 2-inches larger than your 12-inch pizza pan. Have your rolling pin and a 12-inch pizza pan ready.

2. Prepare your double boiler. A sauce pot partially filled with water with your mixing bowl that fits on top will suffice. Over high heat, bring your water in the pot to a simmer, then turn the heat to low.

3. In your mixing bowl for the double boiler. Place your bowl over the simmering pot and stir constantly being careful not to burn yourself with the steam escaping between your pan and the pot. A silicone mitt works well to hold the bowl.

4. Knead for a few minutes to mix your dough thoroughly. Roll your dough into a ball, then place onto the center of your parchment paper. Pat into a disk shape and cover with the other piece of paper. Using your rolling pin, gently roll your dough into about a 12-inch circle.

5. Place your dough and the bottom piece of your parchment onto the pizza pan. Using your fork, poke holes all over the dough. Place your pan in the oven and bake for approximately 6 to 8 minutes, watching carefully. Remove when it is golden brown. Decrease your oven setting to 350 degrees.

6. Spread cheese on flatbread. Arrange your onion slices. Add your apple slices. Layer on your ham pieces. Cover with your remaining 3/4 cup of cheese. Sprinkle with your thyme, salt, and ground pepper. Bake at 350 degrees until your cheese is melted and the crust is golden brown. Should take about 5 to 7 minutes.

7. Remove your apple and ham flatbread from your oven and slide off of the parchment. Transfer to your cutting board and slice it into eight pieces.

Serve!

Nutritional Value

255 Calories.
16 grams of Protein.
4 grams of Carbs.
20 grams of Fat.

47. Broccoli Chicken Zucchini Boats

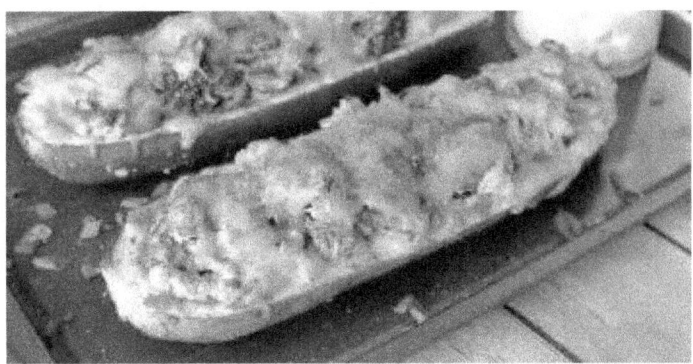

Serving size: This recipe yields 2 servings.

Ingredients

- 6 ounces of Shredded Rotisserie Chicken
- 3 ounces of Shredded Cheddar Cheese
- 2 Large Zucchini (Hollowed Out)
- 2 tablespoons of Sour Cream
- 2 tablespoons of Butter
- One stalk of Green Onion
- 1 cup of Broccoli

- Salt
- Pepper

Directions

1. Preheat your oven to 400 degrees and cut your zucchini in half lengthwise. The longer the zucchini, the better for this specific recipe. Using your spoon, scoop out most of the zucchini until you're left with a shell about 1 centimeter thick.

2. Pour one tablespoon of melted butter into each zucchini boat. Season with your salt and pepper and place them in your oven. It allows your zucchini to cook down while you prepare the filling. This should take approximately 20 minutes.

3. Measure out 6 ounces and save the rest for another meal. Combine your chicken and broccoli with your sour cream to keep them moist and creamy. Season in this step as well. Once your zucchini has had a chance to cook, take them out and add your chicken and broccoli filling.

4. Add cheese your chicken and broccoli and pop them back into your oven for an additional 10 to 15 minutes or until your cheese is melted and browning. Garnish with your chopped green onion and enjoy with sour cream or mayo if so desired. Serve!

Nutritional Value

476 Calories.
30 grams of Protein.
5 grams of Carbs.
34 grams of Fat.

48. Bacon, Avocado, & Chicken Sandwich

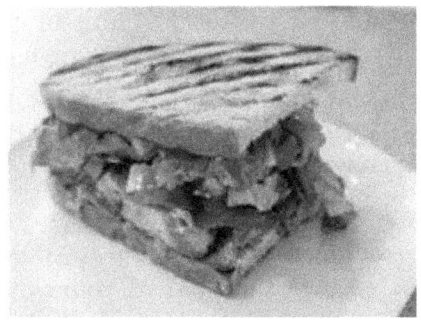

Serving size: This recipe yields 2 servings.

Ingredients

- 3 Large Eggs
- 1/8 teaspoon of Cream of Tartar
- 3 ounces of Cream Cheese
- 1/2 teaspoon of Garlic Powder
- 1/4 teaspoon of Salt

Ingredients for the Filling

- 3 ounces of Chicken
- One tablespoon of Mayonnaise
- Two slices of Pepper Jack Cheese
- One teaspoon of Sriracha
- 1/4 Medium Avocado
- Two slices of Bacon
- 2 Grape Tomatoes

Directions

1. Preheat your oven to 300 degrees. Begin separating your three eggs into to 2 dry bowls. Add your cream of tartar and salt to your egg whites. Using an electric mixer, whip your egg whites until you see soft, foamy peaks form.

2. In your other bowl, combine 3 ounces of cubed cream cheese with your egg yolks and beat until a pale-yellow color. Gently fold your egg whites into your eggs, half at a time. On your parchment paper lined baking sheet, spoon about 1/4 cup of your bread batter.

3. Using your spatula, press gently on tops of the bread to form squares. Then sprinkle the tops with your garlic powder and bake for approximately 25 minutes. While your bread is baking, cook your chicken and bacon with some salt and pepper.

4. To arrange your sandwich, begin by combining mayo and sriracha and spreading that onto the underside of one piece of bread. Add your chicken to your mayo mixture. Add two slices of pepper jack cheese and the bacon.

Nutritional Value

361 Calories.
22 grams of Protein.
2 grams of Carbs.
28 grams of Fat.

49. Simple Chicken Salad

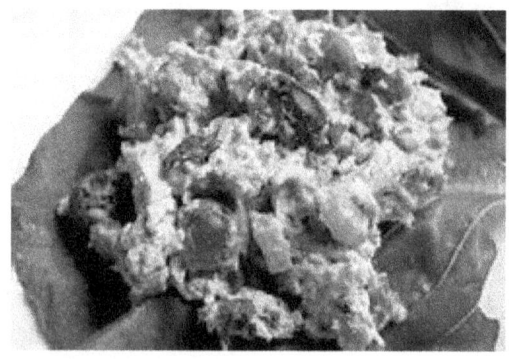

Serving size: This recipe yields 6 servings.

Ingredients

- 4 Chicken Breasts
- 3 Large Hardboiled Eggs
- 3.5 ounces of Green Peppers
- 1 ounce of Green Onions
- 4.5 ounces of Celery
- 3/4 cup of Sugar-Free Sweet Relish
- 3/4 cup of Mayo

Directions

1. Preheat your oven to 350 degrees. Add your chicken to your oven safe pan. Cook for approximately 45 to 60 minutes until your chicken is finished cooking. Place 3 eggs in your pan and cover them with water. Add celery and peppers.

2. Once your chicken is out of your oven allow it to cool down and then chop up. Combine all of your ingredients in your large-sized bowl. Chop up your eggs and mix in. Add your eggs last. Split into six separate portions or containers. Serve!

Nutritional Value

413 Calories.
43 grams of Protein.
2 grams of Carbs.
25 grams of Fat.

50. Easy Buffalo Wings

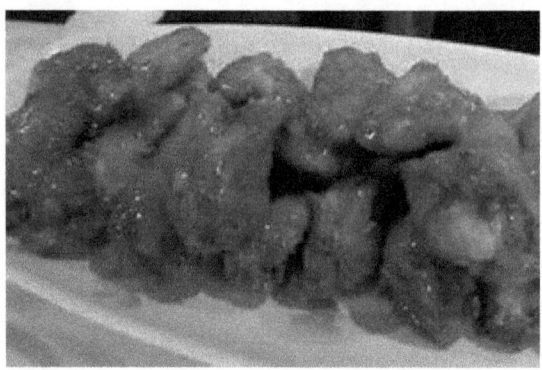

Serving size: This recipe yields 2 servings.

Ingredients

- 6 Chicken Wings (6 Drumettes & 6 Wingettes)
- 1/2 cup of Frank's Red Hot Sauce
- 2 tablespoons of Butter
- Garlic Powder
- Paprika
- Salt
- Pepper
- Cayenne (optional)

Directions

1. Break each of your chicken wings into 2 different pieces. The drumettes and wingettes, getting rid of the tips. Pour your hot sauce over your wings. Enough to lightly coat them. Season your wings with spices and cover them. Place in your refrigerator for 1 hour.

2. Set your broiler on high and put your oven rack 6-inches from your broiler. Place your aluminum paper on your baking sheet. Place your arms on your sheet with enough room so the flames can reach their sides.

3. Cook for approximately 8 minutes under your broiler. Your wings should turn dark brown on top. May turn black if they are close to the flame. Melt your butter on your oven top and add the rest of your hot sauce. Can also add cayenne if you want your wings to be spicier.

4. Once your butter has melted take off of the heat. Get your arms from the broiler and flip them. Cook another 6 to 8 minutes. Once good and browned on all sides take out of your broiler and add to your bowl. Pour butter-hot sauce mixture over your wings. Toss wings to coat evenly. Serve!

Nutritional Value

620 Calories.
48 grams of Protein.
1 gram of Carbs.
46 grams of Fat.

51. Oopsie Rolls

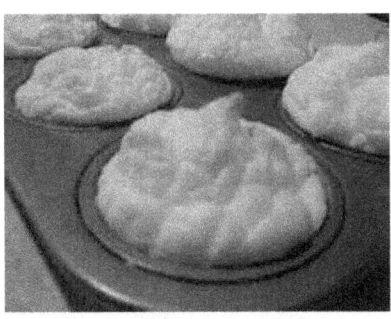

Serving size: This recipe yields 12 servings.

Ingredients

- 3 Large Eggs
- 3 ounces of Cream Cheese

Directions

1. Preheat your oven to 300 degrees. Separate your eggs from egg yolks. Place each in different bowls. With an electric hand, mixer beat your egg whites until they get very bubbly. Add in your cream of tarter. Beat it until a stiff peak has formed.

2. In your egg yolk bowl, add your 3 ounces of cream cheese and salt. Beat your egg yolk mixture until your yolks are a pale looking yellow and they have doubled in their size. Don't use an electric hand mixer. Gently fold it together.

3. Spray with some oil or grease. Dollop your battery as big as you want them. I make 12 of equal size and the nutritional value amount reflects that. Bake for approximately 30 to 40 minutes. They are done when the tops of your oopsie rolls are firm and golden. Allow them to cool on your wire rack. Serve!

Nutritional Value

45 Calories.
2.3 grams of Protein.
0 grams of Carbs.
3.8 grams of Fat.

52. Cucumber Sushi Rolls

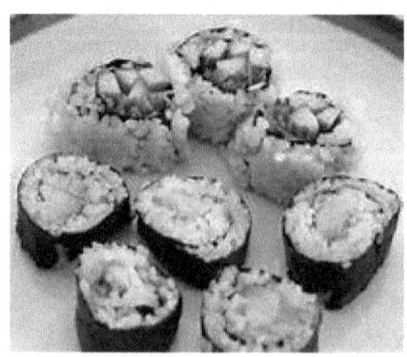

Serving size: This recipe yields 2 servings.

Ingredients

- 1/2 pound of Tuna Steak
- 1/2 Avocado
- 2 Cucumbers
- 2 tablespoons of Mayonnaise
- 8 Shrimp
- 1 stalk of Green Onion

Directions

1. Peel your cucumbers and cut off their ends. You want to have two 6 to 8-inch long cylindrical shaped cucumbers when done. Use your long, wet knife and lay the edge of it against a side of your cucumber. Begin cutting into it. The knife should be barely visible under your thin cucumber. Gather your other ingredients.

2. Mix your mayo and sriracha to make spicy mayo. Take the end of your cucumber with your fish and begin rolling it onto itself. Make sure to keep your roll tight so that no air pockets form. The ingredients need to stick to one another, otherwise, they'll fall right out.

3. Once you're almost done rolling it and only have approximately 2 to 3-inches left of your cucumber, spread some of your spicy mayo on your cucumber and finish the roll. The mayonnaise will act as sort of glue to help keep your cucumber sealed. Carefully slice your cucumber into 1/2 inch to 1-inch rounds. Hold both sides of your cucumber as slicing to help maintain its shape. You should now have 6 to 8 pieces of sushi per roll. Chop up your green onion and sprinkle on top. Serve!

Nutritional Value

322 Calories.

36 grams of Protein.
2.5 grams of Carbs.
17 grams of Fat.

53. Tuna Tartare

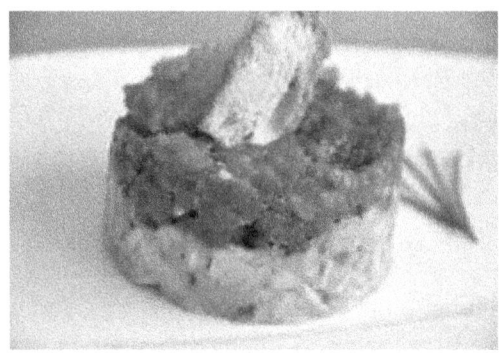

Serving size: This recipe yields 2 servings.

Ingredients

- 1 pound of Tuna Steak
- 1 Avocado
- Three stalks of Scallion
- One teaspoon of Jalapeno
- Sesame Seeds
- 1 tablespoon of Mayo
- 1 tablespoon of Sriracha
- 2 Persian Cucumbers
- 1/2 Lime

Directions

1. Dice your tuna steak and your avocado into 1/4-inch cubes. Put them in your bowl. Dice your jalapeno and scallion. Add them to your bowl.

2. Pour your sesame oil, olive oil, soy sauce, mayo, juice from a lime, and sriracha into your bowl. Gently combine your ingredients using your hands. Slice your Persian cucumber and sprinkle with your sesame seeds. Serve!

Nutritional Value

487 Calories.
56.7 grams of Protein.
4 grams of Carbs.
24.5 grams of Fat.

54. Simple Cucumber Sandwich

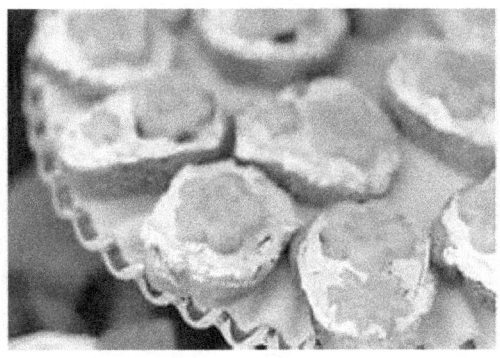

Serving size: This recipe yields 1 serving.

Ingredients

- 1 Cucumber
- 1.5 ounces of Boursin Cheese
- Sliced Meat

Directions

1. Slice your cucumber into half and use your melon to remove any seeds and some of the cucumber itself.

2. Fill the one side with your spreadable Boursin cheese. Fold your sliced deli meat longways so you can fill the other half. Serve!

Nutritional Value (Will Depend on Type of Deli Meat Used)

196 Calories.
17 grams of Protein.
7 grams of Carbs.
12 grams of Fat.

55. Southern Pork Stew

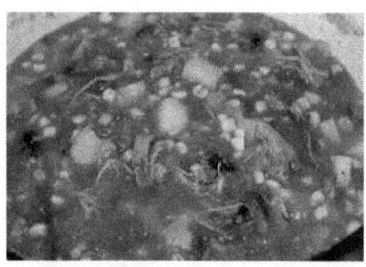

Those midday slumps can certainly put the rest of your day on a slippery slide. We're tired, we're getting hungry, and during the winter months, the feeling to crawl under a blanket for a nap can be almost overwhelming. But fear not! We have the perfect dish that will put some warmth in your belly and a spring in your step. Ready? Well here we go.

Serving size: You'll get four servings.

Ingredients for the Spices

- One tsp. oregano
- One tsp. Paprika
- ¼ tsp. cinnamon
- One tsp. Minced garlic
- Two tsp. cumin
- tsp. chilli powder
- 2 bay leaves

- Salt and pepper to taste (approx ½ tsp. each)

Ingredients for the Meat

- 1 lb. cooked pork shoulder (sliced)

Ingredients for the Vegetables

- ½ green bell pepper (sliced)
- ½ red bell pepper (Sliced)
- ½ medium onion
- 6 oz. button mushrooms
- ½ jalapeno (sliced)

Ingredients for the Soup

- ¼ cup tomato paste
- 2 cups chicken broth
- 2 cups gelatinous bone broth

Ingredients for the Juice

- ½ lime
- ½ cup coffee (your remedy for the midday slump)

Directions

1. Clean and slice all your vegetables. Turn to high heat. Sauté your vegetables until they are just beginning to cook and filling your kitchen with their fantastic aroma. Be careful not to overcook them here! That will give you a slightly mushy stew later on. Set your slow cooker on low; add the bone broth, coffee, and chicken broth.

2. While your slow cooker is warming, add spices and bay leaves to a single bowl. This is a handy step for almost any

recipe and will help you keep all your spices in one place. Now add all your mushrooms and sliced pork to the slow cooker.

3. Give your cooking vegetables and oil a final stir, and add them to the crock pot along with all your spices. Cover, and let the slow cooker work its magic for about 4-10 hours. Once it's finished, remove the bay leaves (or keep an eye out for them), and serve!

Nutritional information (per serving)

Calories: 386
Fat: 29g
Carbs: 6.5g
Protein: 19.8g

56. Keto Bacon Chicken Sandwich with Avocado

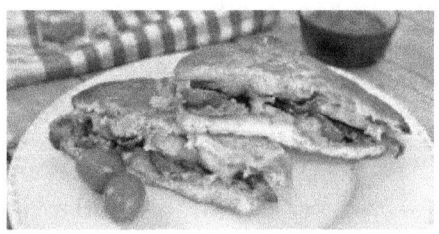

Sandwiches are no longer off limits on the keto diet! Make your bread using egg and cream cheese to keep the fat and protein content up, and top it with cheese and avocado!

Serving size: The recipe yields 2 servings.

Ingredients for the Bread

- 1/4 tsp. salt
- 1/2 tsp. garlic powder
- 1/8 tsp. cream of tartar

- Three large eggs
- 3 oz. cream cheese

Ingredients for the Filling

- 3 oz. chicken
- Two slices bacon
- Two slices pepper jack cheese
- One tsp. sriracha
- 1 tbsp. mayonnaise
- 2 grape tomatoes
- 1/4 avocado

Directions

1. Preheat oven to 300F. Separate your eggs into different bowls. Add cream of tartar and salt to the eggs whites, and whip until you get soft peaks. Add cream cheese to the egg yolks bowl and beat until a smooth pale-yellow color form. Fold the egg white mixture into the yolks. Gently complete this as we want to the whites nice and airy.

2. Line a baking sheet with parchment paper, and pour about 1/4 cup of your bread mixture into individual areas, and form into square shapes. Sprinkle garlic atop the bread and bake for 25 minutes. While the bread is baking, cook the chicken and bacon with a little salt and pepper. Once everything is cooked, assemble your sandwich with the mayo, avocado, cheese, and tomatoes. Enjoy!

Nutritional Information (per serving)

Calories: 355
Fat: 28g
Carbs: 1.5g
Protein: 24g

Enjoying this book?

Check out my other best sellers!

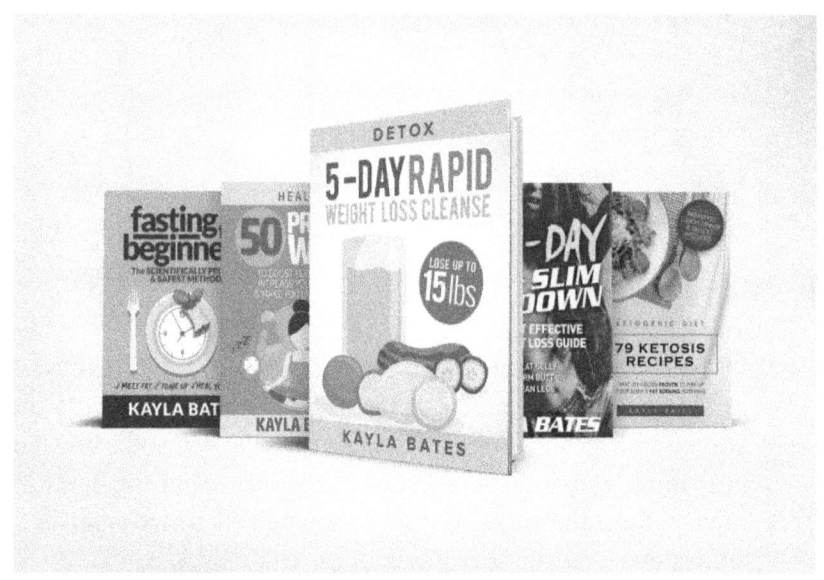

Get your next book on sale here:

TopFitnessAdvice.com/go/Kayla

57. Spring Salad

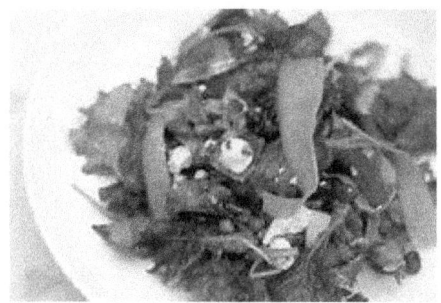

Enjoy this light and sweet salad to keep you going for the afternoon. Bacon and pine nuts will help fill you up while the raspberry vinaigrette gives a distinctly sweet flavor.

Serving size: This recipe yields one serving.

Ingredients

- 2 tbsp. parmesan (shaved)
- 2 tbsp. raspberry vinaigrette
- 2 oz. mixed greens
- 3 tbsp. pine nuts (roasted)
- Two slices bacon
- Salt and pepper to taste

Directions

1. Cook the bacon in a stovetop pan. Beautiful and crispy is what we're aiming for here! Assemble your salad with the rest of the ingredients and crumble the bacon overtop. Shake well to make sure everything in combined. Enjoy!

Nutritional Information (per serving)

Calories: 470
Fat: 36g

Carbs: 4g
Protein: 17.5g

58. Chicken Egg Soup

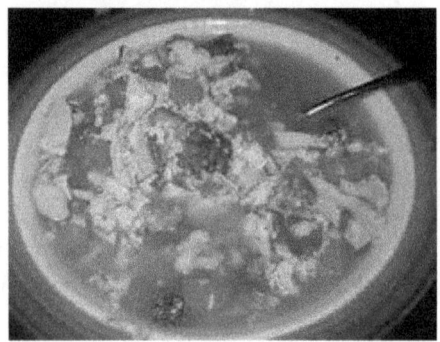

Easy and delicious lunchtime soup! Chicken broth and eggs yield a very savory dish while the incredibly easy preparation makes it the perfect choice for a quick lunch.

Serving size: This recipe yields 1 serving.

Ingredients

- Two large eggs
- 1 tbsp. bacon fat
- One tsp. Chili garlic paste
- 1/2 cube chicken bouillon
- 1 1/2 cups chicken broth

Directions

1. Heat a pan on medium-high, and add the broth, bacon fat, and bouillon cube. Once the soup begins to boil, add the chili paste and stir continually for a minute. Now remove from heat. Beat the eggs in a separate container, and pour in the broth. Serve and enjoy!

Nutritional Information (per serving)

Calories: 275
Fat: 24g
Carbs: 2g
Protein: 13g

59. Jalapeno Mug Cake

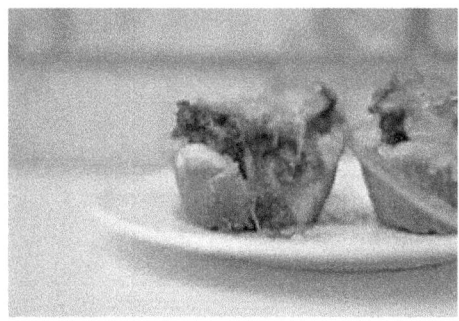

Missing out on lunch is a recipe for a disastrous afternoon. But even on the tightest of schedules, a quick mug cake can still get you a filling lunch! Here we have a zesty jalapeno mug cake made of egg and almond flour.

Serving size: This recipe yields 1 serving.

Ingredients

- One large egg
- 1 tbsp. cream cheese
- 1 tbsp. butter
- 1 slice bacon
- 1/2 tsp. baking powder
- One/2 jalapeno pepper
- 2 tbsp. almond flour
- 1 tbsp. golden flaxseed meal
- 1/4 tsp. salt

Directions

1. Heat a pan over medium, and cook the bacon until nice and crisp. Now in a mug, mix all of the remaining ingredients. Scrape down the sides, so everything is in the bottom of the cup. Microwave for 80 seconds on high.

2. Flip the mug upside down and gently tap against a plate to make the cake fall out, and garnish with the bacon and any leftover jalapenos. Enjoy!

Nutritional information (per serving)

Calories: 430
Fat: 36g
Carbs: 5g
Protein: 16g

60. Enchilada Soup

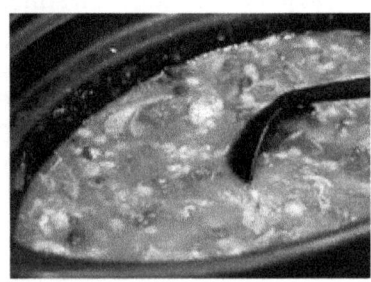

This rich soup will certainly spice up your lunchtime! Chicken, cheese, and a little cayenne pepper will keep you running and on the keto diet at the same time.

Serving size: The recipe yields 4 servings.

Ingredients

- 8 oz. cream cheese

- 4 cups chicken broth
- 6 oz. chicken (shredded)
- 4 stalks celery (diced)
- One red bell pepper (diced)
- 3 tbsp. olive oil
- 1/2 tsp. cayenne pepper
- 1/2 lime (juiced)
- Two tsp. cumin
- One tsp. Chili powder
- 1 tsp. oregano
- 2 tsp. garlic
- 1 cup tomatoes (diced)
- 1/2 cup cilantro (chopped)

Directions

1. Once hot, add the celery and pepper. Once the celery is soft, toss in your tomatoes and cook until they begin to release their juice. Add all your spices to the pan, and stir several times to incorporate. Now add your cilantro and chicken broth to the pot, and crank up the heat to bring to a boil. Simmer for 25 minutes.

2. Now add your cream cheese and again bring to a boil, then reduce heat, then simmer again for 30 minutes. Add the shredded chicken to the pot as well as the lime juice. Stir several times to make sure everything is well mixed. All set! Feel free to garnish with some cilantro or more cheese!

Nutritional information (per serving)

Calories: 350
Fat: 30g
Carbs: 5g
Protein: 14g

61. Keto Pepper and Basil Pizza

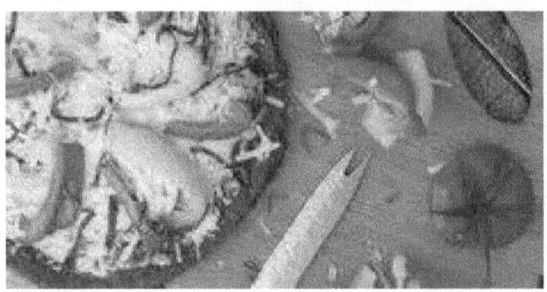

Lose the carb filled flour behind and swap in almond meal for the crust to this delicious lunchtime pizza. Keep it light with peppers and basil or pile on the meat, either way this is a keto friendly dish!

Serving size: This recipe yields two servings (1/2 of one pizza).

Ingredients for the Crust

- 1 large egg
- 2 tbsp. cream cheese
- 2 tbsp. psyllium husk
- 1 tsp. Italian seasoning
- 2 tbsp. parmesan cheese
- 6 oz. mozzarella cheese
- 1/2 cup almond flour
- 1/2 tsp. each of salt and pepper

Ingredients for the Toppings

- 1/4 cup tomato sauce
- 3 tbsp. fresh basil (chopped)
- 4 oz. cheddar cheese (shredded)
- 2/3 bell pepper
- 1 vine tomato

Directions

1. Preheat your oven to 400F. Give your mozzarella (for the crust) a quick 45-second zap in the microwave to melt it. Add all the other crust ingredients to the cheese and mix together completely.

2. Use your hands, or a rolling pin, to flatten the dough and make a circle. Bake this for 10 minutes, and remove from the oven. Now throw on all your toppings, and bake for an additional 10 minutes. Remove pizza and let it cool. It's all yours!

Nutritional information (per serving)

Calories: 420
Fat: 30g
Carbs: 6g
Protein: 25g

62. Breezy Caprese Salad

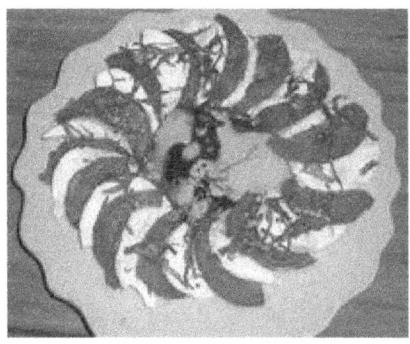

Piles and piles of tomatoes, mozzarella and basil, what could be better? This simple lunch is delicious and filling, especially for those cheese hounds out there.

Serving size: The recipe yields two servings.

Ingredients

- 3 tbsp. olive oil
- 6 oz. mozzarella cheese
- 1 tomato
- 1/4 cup fresh basil (chopped)
- Black pepper and salt to taste

Directions

1. Use a blender, or food processor, to pulse the basil and olive oil. It will leave you will a basil paste. Now slice your tomato into about 1/4 "slices. We're looking for six slices here, so feel free to grab another tomato if you need to!

2. Cut the mozzarella into 1 oz. Slices (right about the same size as the tomatoes or slightly thicker). Layer your Caprese with the tomato as the base, then cheese, and topped with basil paste. Season with salt and pepper to taste. Dig in! Feel free to garnish with extra olive oil.

Nutritional Information (per serving)

Calories: 406
Fat: 35g
Carbs: 5g
Protein: 17g

63. Keto Peanut Shrimp Curry

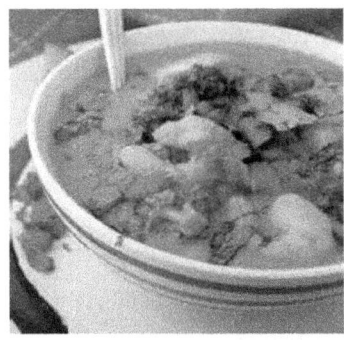

No need to stick to the hurried, unsatisfying, lunches we're used to. Give things a unique twist with this dish featuring shrimp and curry!

Serving size: This recipe yields two servings.

Ingredients

- One tsp. Fish sauce
- 1 tbsp. peanut butter
- 1 tsp. ginger (minced)
- 1 tsp. roasted garlic (crushed)
- 1 tbsp. soy sauce
- 1/4 tsp. xanthan gum
- 1/2 tsp. turmeric
- 3 tbsp. cilantro (chopped)
- 2 tbsp. coconut oil
- 1 spring onion (chopped)
- 1 cup vegetable stock
- 1/2 cup sour cream
- 1 cup coconut milk
- 5 oz. broccoli florets
- 2 tbsp. green curry paste
- 6 oz. shrimp (cooked)
- 1/2 lime (juiced)

Directions

1. When hot, toss in the garlic, spring onion, and ginger. Stir for a few minutes; and once cooked, add 1 tbsp. Of the green curry paste. Along with your soy sauce, turmeric, peanut butter and fish sauce. Continue to stir and cook for several minutes.

2. Add the xanthan gum, and mix completely. Continue to stir, and add the cilantro. Lastly; add the shrimp and mix everything up. Allow it to cook for a few more minutes to allow the shrimp taste to develop. Serve with your sour cream on top and enjoy!

Nutritional information (per serving)

Calories: 450
Fat: 32g
Carbs: 8.5g
Protein: 28g

64. Cucumber Salad

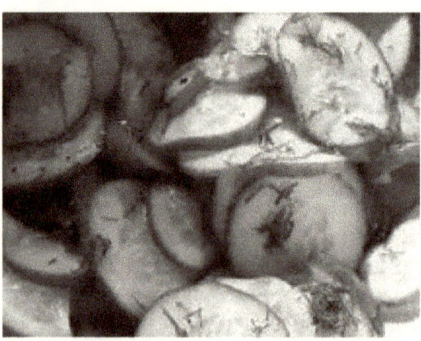

Just like a mug cake, a salad can be the quick and easy solution to a hectic midday. Throw this cucumber salad together in mere minutes and enjoy the combination of noodles and cucumber.

Serving size: This recipe yields one serving.

Ingredients

- 1/4 tsp. red pepper flakes
- 1 tbsp. rice vinegar
- 1 tbsp. sesame oil
- 1 tsp. sesame seeds
- 2 tbsp. olive oil
- One spring onion
- 1 packet shirataki noodles
- 3/4 large cucumber
- salt and pepper to taste

Directions

1. Thoroughly rinse and wash your shirataki noodles, and allow them to dry on a paper towel. Heat a pan over medium-high, and add the coconut oil. Once the pan is hot, add your noodles and fry them for 6 minutes. They should shrink a great deal and any extra liquid will boil off. Remove the noodles from the pan and again set them on a paper towel to dry.

2. Slice the cucumber into whatever sized slices you want, and arrange over a plate. Now top the cucumber with all the other ingredients (other than the noodles), and set in the fridge for 30 minutes. Remove from the fridge, top with the noodles, and serve. Enjoy!

Nutritional information (per serving)

Calories: 415
Fat: 44g
Carbs: 6g
Protein: 2g

65. Ginger Glazed Salmon

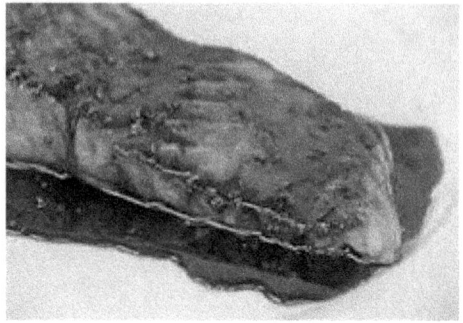

This real ginger covered salmon is sure to put a smile on your face. A quick recipe with a delicious combination of spices, this is sure to become a lunchtime favorite.

Serving size: This recipe yields two servings.

Ingredients

- 1 tbsp. red boat fish sauce
- 2 tsp. garlic (minced)
- 1 tbsp. ketchup (sugar-free)
- One tsp. Ginger (minced)
- 1 tbsp. rice vinegar
- 2 tbsp. white wine
- 2 tbsp. soy sauce
- 2 tsp. sesame oil
- 10 oz. salmon fillet

Directions

1. Toss all of your ingredients except for the ketchup, white wine, and sesame oil into a container. Let these marinate for about 15 minutes. Heat a pan on high and add the sesame oil. As soon as the oil lets off a little smoke, add the fish with the skin side down.

2. Allow the fish skin to crisp up and cook, then flip and continue cooking. It takes about 3 to 4 minutes per side. After the first flip,

add all the marinade ingredients to the pan and let them cook with the fish.

3. When cooked, remove the salmon from the pan. Add the ketchup and white wine to the liquid left in the pan. Let everything simmer for 6 minutes, and put inside the dish. Serve it up with the sauce on the side.

Nutritional information (per serving)

Calories: 375
Fat: 22g
Carbs: 2g
Protein: 34g

66. Keto Tomato Pesto Mug Cake

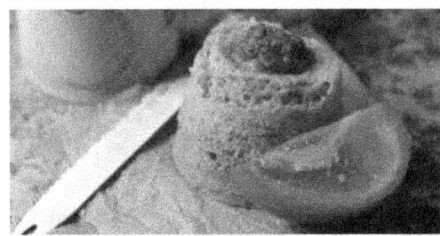

Another mug cake recipe for those hectic lunches! This tomato and pesto filled cake is tasty and would make an excellent addition to some Caprese salad!

Serving size: The recipe yields one serving.

Ingredients

- 2 tbsp. butter
- 2 tbsp. almond flour
- One large egg
- 1/2 tsp. baking powder

Ingredients for the Pesto

- 1 tbsp. almond flour
- Five tsp. sun dried tomato pesto
- 1 pinch salt

Directions

1. Combine all ingredients in a mug (keep some pesto in reserve if you want it as a topping). Microwave the mug on high for 70 to 80 seconds. Lightly tap the mug against a plate, and the mug will fall out. Top with any leftover pesto. Quick and easy, enjoy!

Nutritional information (per serving)

Calories: 460
Fat: 45g
Carbs: 4g
Protein: 13g

67. Keto Cabbage Rolls with Corned Beef

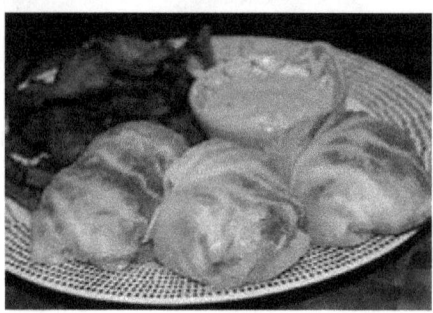

These corned beef cabbage rolls are delicious, filling, and make a wonderful presentation if you're entertaining. The subtle hint of cloves and allspice provide an excellent finish to this dish!

Serving size: This recipe yields five servings:

Ingredients

- 1 tbsp. erythritol
- 1 tbsp. bacon fat
- One fresh lemon
- 1 tbsp. brown mustard
- 1 tsp. whole peppercorns
- 2 tsp. Worcestershire sauce
- 1 tsp. mustard seeds
- 1/4 tsp. cloves
- 1/4 allspice
- 1/2 tsp. red pepper flakes
- 2 tsp. salt
- 1/4 cup coffee
- 1 medium onion
- 1/4 cup white wine
- 15 large cabbage leaves
- 1.5 lbs. corned beef
- 1 bay leaf (crushed)

Directions

1. In a slow cooker, combine all your spices, liquids, and the corned beef. Turn the slow cooker to low, and leave for 6 hours. When ready, bring a pot of water to boiling, and add all cabbage leaves as well as the sliced onion. After 3 minutes remove the cabbage leaves, and dump them in some ice water for a further 4 minutes. Remember the onions should still be in the boiling water!

2. Slice the meat and dry off the cabbage leaves. Remove the onion from the water. All the fillings into each cabbage leaf, and give a squirt of lemon juice overtop for good measure. Enjoy!

Nutritional information (per serving)

Calories: 475

Fat: 27g
Carbs: 4g
Protein: 34.5g

68. Keto Sausage Pepper Soup

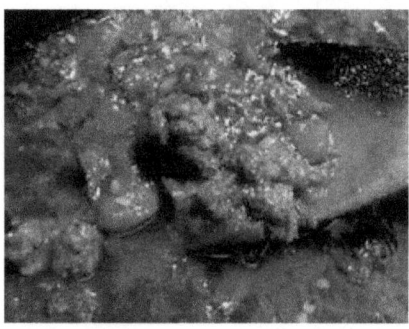

This hearty soup is perfect for a drizzly lunchtime. It will leave your house, or office, with a pleasant aroma and the addition of hot sausage and jalapenos, are sure to give you a kick!

Serving size: This recipe yields 4 servings.

Ingredients

- Two tsp. Chili powder
- 2 tsp. garlic (minced)
- 2 tsp. cumin
- One tsp. Italian seasoning
- 1 green bell pepper
- 6 cups raw spinach
- 1/2 medium onion
- One can eat tomatoes with jalapenos
- 1.4 lbs. hot Italian sausage
- 2 cups beef stock
- 1/2 tsp. salt
- 1 red bell pepper

Directions

1. Tear the sausage into chunks and cook on the stove until fully cooked. Slice your peppers; and add them, tomatoes, all spices, and beef stock to a crock pot. Top the crock pot with the sausage and mix.

2. Fry your onions and garlic until the garlic begins to brown. Top with the spinach. Cook for 3 hours. After 3 hours, open it up and give everything a stir, then cook a further 2 hours. Serve it up!

Nutritional Information (per serving)

Calories: 380
Fat: 28g
Carbs: 7g
Protein: 25g

69. Coconut Curry

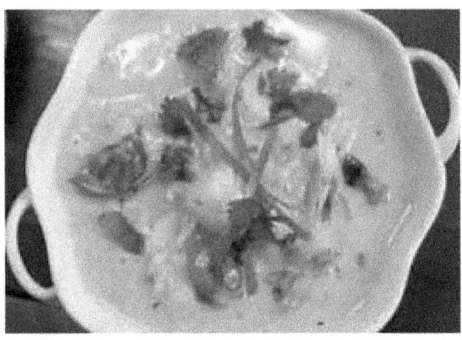

Would all the coconut lovers please stand up. We hope that includes most of you because this fantastic combination of curry and coconut is certain to give your lunch hour a zing!

Serving size: This recipe yields 2 servings.

Ingredients

- Two tsp. red boat fish sauce
- One tsp. garlic (minced)
- 2 tsp. soy sauce
- 1 tsp. ginger (minced)
- 4 tbsp. coconut oil
- 1 cup broccoli florets
- 1 tbsp. red curry paste
- 1/4 onion
- One large handful spinach

Directions

1. Add 2 tbsp. Coconut oil to a pan on medium-high. Put the garlic in the pan. When the garlic begins to brown, turn heat down to medium, and add broccoli. Stir everything together, and when the broccoli is partially cooked, move everything to one side of the pan. Add the curry paste to the open aspect of the pan, and let cook for 60 seconds.

2. Now toss the spinach on top of the broccoli until it begins to wilt, then add the coconut cream and rest of the oil. Stir everything together, and add the fish sauce, ginger, and soy sauce. Let simmer for 10 minutes. Enjoy!

Nutrition information (per serving)

Calories: 395
Fat: 40g
Carbs: 7g
Protein: 6g

70. Keto Turkey Meatballs

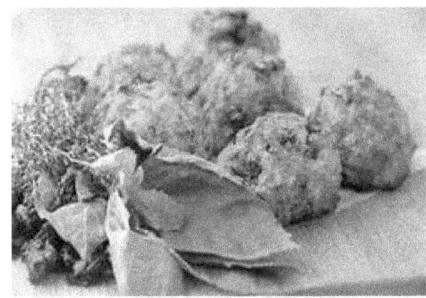

If it's a 'plate of meatballs all to myself' kind of day, or if you're in charge of appetizers for a party, these keto friendly turkey meatballs are just the ticket!

Serving size: This recipe yields 20 servings/meatballs.

Ingredients

- 1/2 salt
- 1/2 pepper
- Three sprigs thyme
- Two large handfuls of spinach
- 3 small red chilies
- Ten slices bacon
- Two lbs. Ground turkey
- 1/2 green pepper
- 2 large eggs
- One oz. Pork rinds
- 1 small onion

Directions

1. Place bacon on top. Preheat oven to 400F. Bake until the desired crispiness is reached. While the bacon is cooking, add all ingredients (except ground turkey and spinach) to a food processor and mince well. Insert the minced mixture to the ground turkey and mix well.

2. Once the bacon is done, drain the fat into an individual container. Now form 20 meatballs from your mixture and place on the same baking sheet that you used before. Cook meatballs for 20 minutes or until the juice begins to run clear.

3. Skewer 2 to 3 pieces of bacon to each meatball. Now in a food processor, blend the spinach, leftover bacon fat, and any spices you wish until you have a paste. Serve the meatballs on top of the paste and enjoy!

Nutritional Information (per serving)

Calories: 140
Fat: 10.5g
Carbs. 0.5g
Protein: 11g

71. Pumpkin Soup

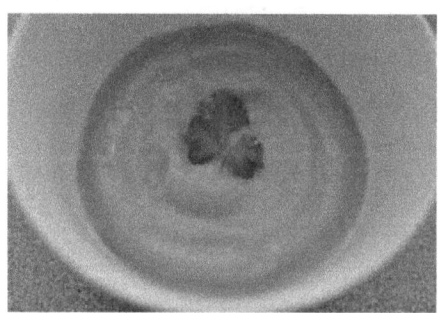

A mellow soup bursting with autumn spice and pumpkin, this soup is perfect for fending off the cold as the seasons change. It's also an excellent remedy for a rainy day!

Serving size: This recipe yields three servings (1 cup each).

Ingredients

- 1/2 tsp. pepper

- 1/2 tsp. salt
- 1/4 tsp. ginger (minced)
- 1/4 tsp. coriander
- 1/8 tsp. nutmeg
- 1/4 tsp. cinnamon
- 2 cloves garlic (roasted and minced)
- 4 tbsp. butter
- 1 cup pumpkin puree
- 1/2 cup heavy cream
- 4 slices bacon
- 1 bay leaf
- 1/4 onion (chopped)
- 3 tbsp. bacon grease
- 1 1/2 cups chicken broth

Directions

1. Add the butter to a saucepan over medium-low heat, and heat until it begins to brown. When the butter is dark golden in color, add your garlic, ginger, and onions. Cook for 3 minutes, and once the onions are translucent, add all of your spices and stir completely. Mix chicken broth and pumpkin. Increase heat and bring to a boil. Once boiling, reduce heat and simmer for 20 minutes.

2. Transfer everything to a blender and puree until smooth or desired consistency. Return to pot and simmer for a further 20 minutes. Now cook your bacon in whatever style you wish. When the soup is ready, add heavy cream and bacon grease. Mix well. Crumble your bacon on top and serve. Savor and enjoy!

Nutritional information (per serving)

Calories: 485
Fat: 47g
Carbs: 7.5g

Protein: 6g

72. Chicken Satay

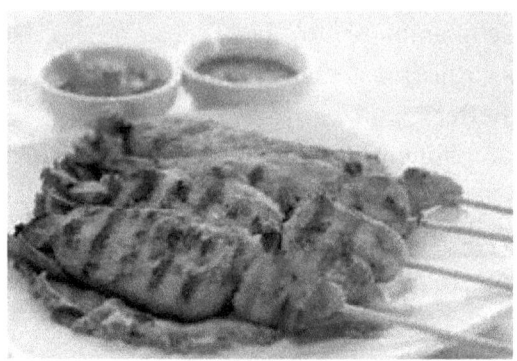

The upbeat combination of cayenne pepper, paprika, and peanut butter this a filling and enjoyable. Furthermore, we've kept the carb countdown to keep you on your keto diet.

Serving size: This recipe yields three servings.

Ingredients

- 1 tbsp. rice vinegar
- Two tsp. Chili paste
- 1/4 tsp. cayenne pepper
- 2 tsp. sesame oil
- 1 tbsp. erythritol
- 1 tsp. garlic (minced)
- 1/4 tsp. paprika
- 1/3 yellow pepper
- 4 tbsp. soy sauce
- 1 lb. ground chicken
- 2 spring onions
- 3 tbsp. peanut butter
- 1/2 lime (juiced)

Directions

1. Place pan over medium-high heat, and add sesame oil. When hot, brown your chicken. Add all other ingredients, except onion and yellow pepper, to the pan and mix well.

2. When everything is cooked all the way through, add your onion and pepper. Continue to cook until onion is translucent. Salt and pepper to taste and serve. Nicely done, enjoy!

Nutritional information (per serving)

Calories: 390
Fat: 22g
Carbs: 3.5g
Protein: 34g

73. Bacon and Cheddar Mug Cake

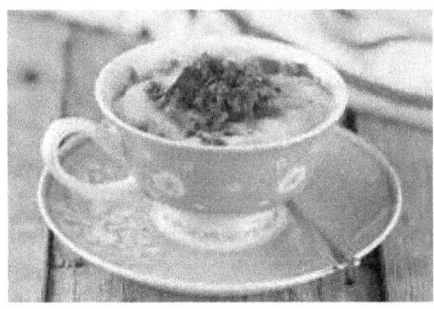

The easy mug cake sure packs a punch! A hot bacon, cheddar, and chive cake that's delicious and only takes a few minutes!

Serving size: This recipe yields 1 serving.

Ingredients for the Base

- 2 tbsp. almond flour
- 1 large egg

- 2 tbsp. butter
- 1/2 tsp. baking powder

Ingredients for the Inner

- 1 tbsp. white cheddar (shredded)
- 1 tbsp. chive (chopped)
- 1 tbsp. cheddar (shredded)
- 2 slices bacon
- 1/4 tsp. Mrs. Dash (table blend)
- 1 tbsp. almond flour
- 1 pinch salt

Directions

1. Mix all your base ingredients together. Stir well, so there are no clumps. Now chop your bacon (already cooked) and chives, and add these two along with all your innards ingredients together. Mix well.

2. Now mix everything together in a mug, and microwave on high for 70 seconds. Lightly tap the mug against a plate and the cake will tumble out. Serve it up! Add extra chives on top if you wish.

Nutritional information (per serving)

Calories: 570
Fat: 54g
Carbs: 6g
Protein: 25g

74. Keto Inside-Out Burger

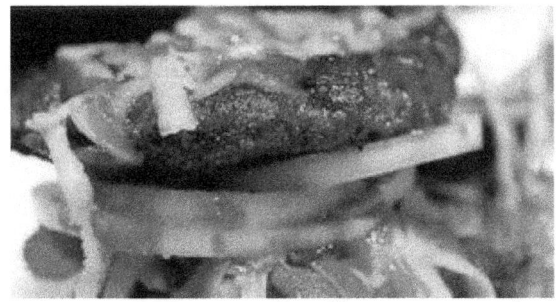

Want to avoid the carbs in a burger? Then just toss out! This inside out burger is delicious and features two patties forming the 'bun' stuffed with all your favorite burger toppings.

Serving size: This recipe yields six servings.

Ingredients

- Eight slices bacon (chopped)
- Two tsp. garlic (minced)
- 28 oz. ground beef
- 2 tbsp. chives (chopped)
- 2 tsp. black pepper
- 1 tbsp. soy sauce
- 1 tsp. Worcestershire sauce
- 1 1/4 tsp. salt
- 1 tsp. onion powder
- 1/4 cup cheddar cheese

Directions

1. Heat up a cast iron skillet and cook your chopped bacon until nice and crispy. Remove to a paper towel once cooked and reserve the grease. In a bowl, mix all of your spices, the ground beef, and 2/3 of the bacon. Mix altogether. Form about nine patties. Now toss about 2 tbsp. of the bacon fat back into the skillet.

2. Once hot and sizzling, add your patties and cook about 5 minutes. Remove the patties from the pan and let them cool for about 5 minutes. Serve them up with cheese, more bacon, and onion if you like. All your favorite burger toppings! Enjoy!

Nutritional Information (per serving)

Calories: 430
Fat: 35g
Carbs: 2g
Protein: 30g

75. Scrumptious Sunday Roast

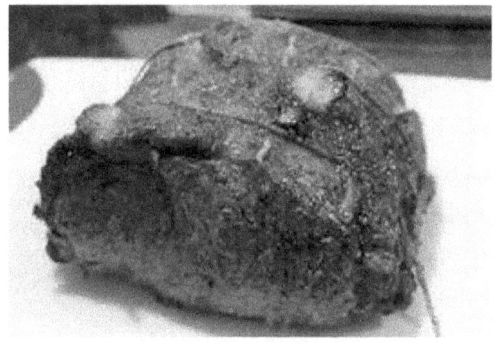

Feeling ambitious for your weekend lunch? Then break out a beef rib roast and get it cooking in your slow cooker all morning, filling your house with a pleasant aroma in the process!

Serving size: This recipe yields eight servings.

Ingredients

- 1 tsp. garlic powder
- Two tsp. salt
- One tsp. pepper
- 5 lbs. beef rib roast

Directions

1. Take your rib roast out of the fridge and let it come to room temperature for about an hour. Preheat your oven to 375F. Break out your roasting rack, or a casserole dish will work as well. Give your roast a rub down with all your spices. Place the roast in whatever oven safe dish you're using, and cook for 1 hour.

2. After 1 hour, turn off the oven, but DO NOT open the door. Let it sit in the turned-off oven for another 3 hours. This will make your roast nice and tender. About 45 minutes prior to serving, turn the oven back on to heat up the roast. After removing from the oven, let the roast rest for about 15 minutes before slicing. Serving with your favorite vegetables and enjoy!

Nutritional information (per serving)

Calories: 680
Fat: 45g
Carbs: 0.5g
Protein: 92g

76. Chicken Stir Fry with Bacon

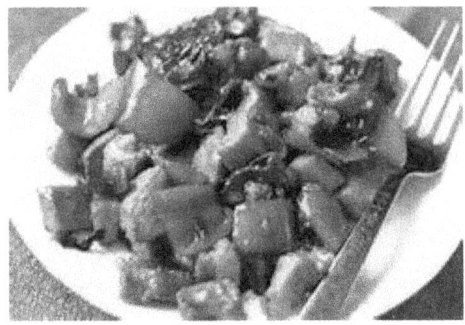

This quick stir-fry features cheesy sausages amongst a pile of vegetables and swimming in a zesty sauce of pepper flakes and butter. Perfect for preparing on the weekend and taking to work throughout the week!

Serving size: This recipe yields 3 servings.

Ingredients

- Two tbsp. butter (salted)
- 1/2 tsp. pepper
- 2 tsp. garlic (minced)
- 1/2 tsp. red pepper flakes
- 1/2 cup parmesan cheese
- 3 cups broccoli florets
- 1/2 cup tomato sauce
- 3 cups spinach
- 1/2 tsp. salt
- 4 cheddar & bacon chicken sausages

Directions

1. Slice your sausage into whatever sizes you wish. Heat a pan on high, and toss in your sausage. Also, bring a separate pot of water to boiling. Throw your broccoli into the boiling water. Cook for about 5 minutes or until it reaches your desired consistency. Continue to stir your sausages as they cook, until they are uniformly brown. Nudge your sausages to one side of the pan and then drop the butter onto the other side.

2. Cut your garlic into the butter and cook for 1 to 2 minutes. Now stir everything in your pan together and add your broccoli as well. Pour the red wine and tomato sauce. Sprinkle the pepper flakes in as well. Mix everything together. Add the spinach, salt, and pepper. Continue to stir as it cooks down. Simmer for 10 minutes. You're all set, enjoy!

Nutritional information (per serving)

Calories: 450
Fat: 29g

Carbs: 8g
Protein: 36g

77. Beefy Stuffed Peppers

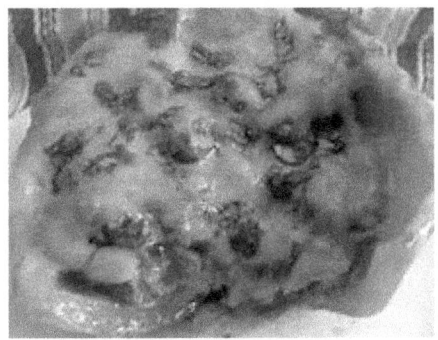

The classic stuffed pepper with beef and bacon! Not a hassle to prepare and excellent for keeping in the fridge for future use.

Serving size: This recipe yields four servings.

Ingredients

- 1 tsp. hot sauce
- 1 tbsp. garlic (minced)
- 1 tsp. liquid smoke
- 3 tbsp. olive oil
- 1 1/2 tsp. Worcestershire sauce
- 1 tbsp. soy sauce
- 2 tsp. oregano
- 1/2 tsp. black pepper
- 2 tbsp. ketchup (sugar free)
- 4 bell peppers
- 1 1/2 lbs. ground beef
- 4 slices bacon (thick cut)

Directions

1. Break out a Ziploc bag, and toss in your meat, spices, and oil. Seal the bag, and mix all the contents thoroughly. Allow this bag to sit in the fridge for at least 3 hours. Preheat your oven to 350F, and bring a pot of salted water to a boil on the stove. Blanch the peppers in the boiling water for 3 minutes, and then immediately remove and dry them.

2. Finely chop your bacon and give it a light fry, don't cook it all the way. Add this bacon to the beef mixture. Now stuff the peppers with the bacon and beef mixture. Bake the peppers for 55 minutes. Sprinkle some cheese on top, and broil until the cheese is bubbling. Serve and enjoy!

Nutritional information (per serving)

Calories: 590
Fat: 42g
Carbs: 5g
Protein: 49g

78. Cheddar Draped Meatballs

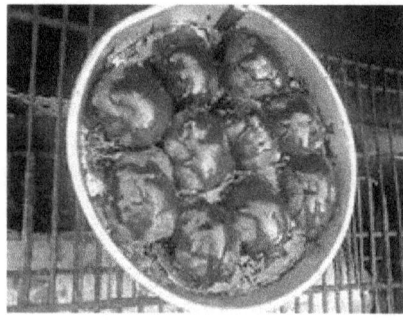

What could make your perfect meatballs even better? Wrap them in a cloak of cheddar cheese! These meatballs are perfect for the main event of your lunch or an appetizer for a party.

Serving size: This recipe yields 24 servings.

Ingredients

- 1 tsp. cumin
- One cup cheddar cheese
- 1 cup tomato sauce
- 1/3 pork rinds (crushed)
- 2 large eggs
- 1 tsp. chili powder
- 1 1/2 chorizo sausage
- 1 1/2 lbs. ground beef
- 1 tsp. salt

Directions

1. Preheat your oven to 350F. Break up your sausage and mix it with the ground beef. You want a relatively uniform mixture here. Now add your pork rinds, spices, cheese, and eggs to the beef mixture. Combine well.

2. Form your meatballs and lay them on a foiled baking sheet. Bake for about 35 minutes, or until thoroughly cooked. Drizzle the tomato sauce over the meatballs and serve. Enjoy!

Nutritional information (per serving)

Calories: 113
Fat: 8g
Carbs: 1g
Protein: 10g

79. Pepper Jack Meatballs

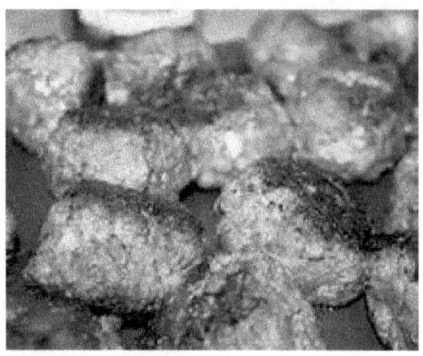

Another fantastic meatball recipe! Here we have pepper jack cheese, Italian sausage, and beef to keep the hunger at bay.

Serving size: This recipe yields 11 servings/meatballs.

Ingredients

- Five slices pepper jack cheese
- One tsp. oregano
- Two large eggs
- One/3 cup pork rinds (crushed)
- 1 cup alfredo sauce
- 1 tsp. Italian seasoning
- 1 1/2 hot Italian sausage.
- 1 1/2 lbs. ground beef
- 1 tsp. salt

Directions

1. Preheat your oven to 350F. Break up the sausage and mix with the meat. Now add the eggs, pork rinds, and spices to the beef mixture. Mix well. Grab about 2/3 of the flesh you would need for each meatball and form into a semicircle.

2. Place the pepper jack cheese on top of the circle and then seal it up with the rest of the meat you need for that meatball. Place the

meatballs on a foiled baking sheet and bake for 40 minutes, or until completely cooked. Drizzle with alfredo sauce and serve. Enjoy!

Nutritional information (per serving)

Calories: 290
Fat: 20g
Carbs: 1.5g
Protein: 23g

80. Bok Choy Salad with Tofu

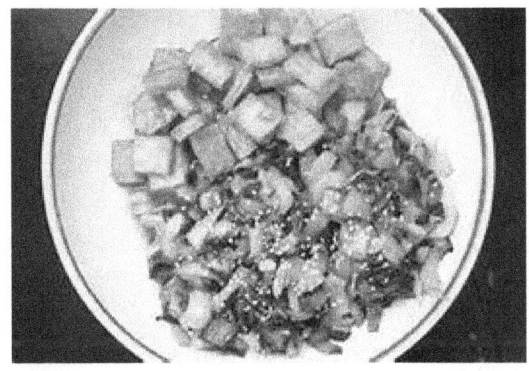

Here we have an interesting twist on the same old lunch salad. Switch things up by using bok choy, a thick leafy green, and cooking your tofu. The tofu will have to be prepared the night before, but it's an excellent and filling lunch!

Serving size: This recipe yields 3 servings.

Ingredients for the Tofu

- 1 tbsp. water
- 1 tbsp. soy sauce
- Two tsp. Garlic (minced)
- 1 tbsp. red wine vinegar

- 1 tbsp. sesame oil
- 15 oz. firm tofu
- 1/2 lemon (juiced)

Ingredients for the Salad

- 1 stalk green onion
- 2 tbsp. soy sauce
- 3 tbsp. coconut oil
- 1 tbsp. sambal look
- 2 tbsp. cilantro (chopped)
- 9 oz. bok choy
- 1 tbsp. peanut butter
- 1/2 lime (juiced)
- 7 drops liquid stevia

Directions

1. Press dry the tofu. It will take nearly 6 hours. Chop the tofu into uniform cubes, and drop into a plastics bag along with the marinade. Let the tofu marinade overnight. Now, preheat your oven to 350F. Place the tofu on a backing sheet (on top of parchment paper), and bake for 35 minutes.

2. While this is baking, mix all the salad ingredients (except the toy). Add the cilantro and spring onion, and mix well. Chop up the bok choy to whatever size you wish and remove the tofu from the oven. Assemble your salad and enjoy!

Nutritional information (per serving)

Calories: 440
Fat: 36g
Carbs: 6g
Protein: 26g

81. Keto Friendly Nasi Lemak

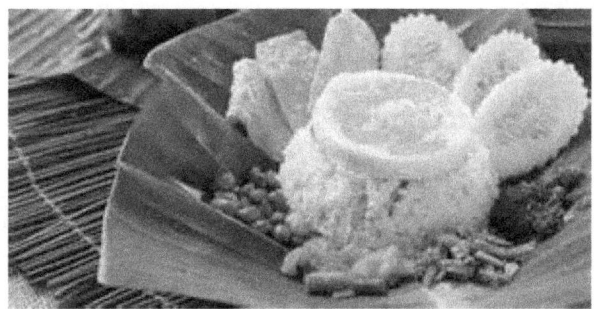

Take an adventure for your lunch and cook up some nasi lemak! This dish consists of rice and chicken cooked in coconut milk and is certain to give you some lunchtime flair!

Serving size: This recipe yields two servings.

Ingredients for the Chicken

- 1/4 tsp. turmeric powder
- 1/8 tsp. salt
- 1/2 tsp. lime juice
- 1/2 tsp. curry powder
- 1/2 tsp. coconut oil
- 2 chicken thighs (boneless)

Ingredients for the Nasi Lemak

- 1/2 small shallot
- 1/4 tsp. salt
- Three slices ginger
- 3 tbsp. coconut milk
- 7 oz. riced cauliflower
- 4 slices cucumber

Ingredients for the Fried Egg

- One large egg
- 1/2 tbsp. butter (unsalted)

Directions

1. Squeeze the water out of your riced cauliflower. Combine your lime juice, salt, turmeric powder, and curry powder. Marinade the chicken thighs with this. Fry the chicken until fully cooked.

2. Heat a saucepan, and toss in ginger, shallot, and coconut milk. Bring to a boil. Once this is boiling, add the cauliflower rice and stir. Fry your egg separately. Dish up your rice mixture and eggs. Serve with two slices of cucumber. All set!

Nutritional information (per serving)

Calories: 502
Fat: 40g
Carbs; 7g
Protein: 29g

Dinner

82. Nutty Salmon

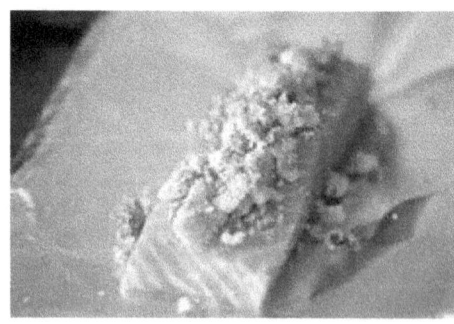

This walnut crust salmon is sure to be a hit for dinner. Deliciously seasoned with mustard and dill, and it's packed with healthy fats to keep you on your diet.

Serving size: This recipe yields two servings.

Ingredients

- 1/4 tsp. dill
- 1 tbsp. olive oil
- 1 tbsp. dion mustard
- Two salmon fillets (3 oz. each)
- 1/2 cup walnuts
- 2 tbsp. maple syrup (sugar-free)
- Salt and pepper to taste

Directions

1. Preheat your oven to 350F. Dump your sugar, mustard, and walnuts into a blender or food processor. Pulse until you have a paste. Heat a stovetop pan on high. Once hot, place your salmon skin side down in the pan. Sear the salmon for about 3 minutes until the skin is crisp.

2. While browning the skin side, add the walnut paste to the side facing up. Once done searing, transfer to the oven and bake for 7 to 8 minutes. All done, enjoy!

Nutritional information (per serving)

Calories: 375
Fat: 44g
Carbs: 4g
Protein: 22g

83. Crock Pot Oxtails

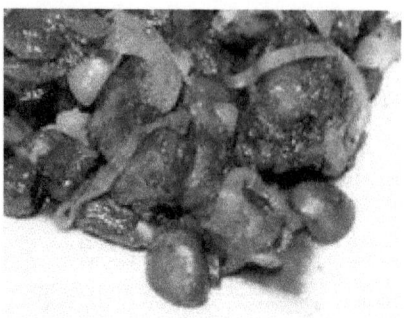

The crock pot is your best friend for dinner on a busy schedule. Just toss in the ingredients, forget for a few hours, and you've got an excellent hot meal already. One such recipe is this crock pot oxtails dish.

Serving size: This recipe yields three servings.

Ingredients

- One tsp. Onion powder
- 3 tbsp. tomato paste
- One tsp. Garlic (minced)
- 1 tbsp. fish sauce
- 2 tbsp. soy sauce
- One tsp. Thyme (dried)
- 1/2 tsp. ginger (ground)
- 1/3 cup butter
- 2 lbs. oxtails
- 2 cups beef broth
- 1/2 tsp. guar gum
- Salt and pepper to taste

Directions

1. Heat the beef broth on the stove, then add the fish sauce, tomato paste, soy sauce, and butter. Once thoroughly cooked and mixed,

add the mixture to a slow cooker and season with all your spices. Insert the oxtails to the slow cooker and mix well. Cook for 7 hours.

2. Remove just the oxtails from the slow cooker, and set aside. Now add the guar gum to what remains in the slow cooker, and use an immersion blender to pulse your mixture. Now serve your oxtails and sauce along with your favorite side dish. Enjoy!

Nutritional information (per serving)

Calories; 430
Fat: 30g
Carbs: 3.5g
Protein: 29g

84. Keto Asian Style Short Ribs

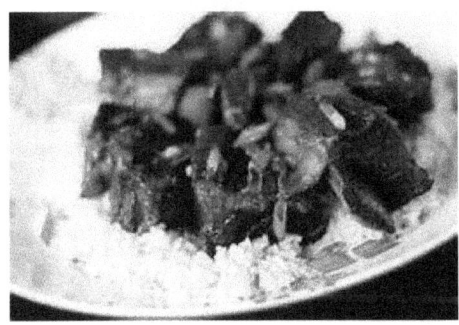

Give your standard ribs a delightful twist by throwing in some Asian style spice! The combination of ginger, soy sauce, and red pepper give this recipe an excellent kick.

Serving size: This recipe yields four servings.

Ingredients for Ribs and Marinade

- 2 tbsp. rice vinegar
- 1/4 cup soy sauce

- 2 tbsp. fish sauce
- Six large short ribs, flank cut (about 1.5 lbs.)

Ingredients for the Asian Spice

- 1/2 tsp. red pepper flakes
- 1/2 tsp. garlic (minced)
- 1/2 tsp. onion powder
- One tsp. Ginger (ground)
- 1/2 tsp. sesame seed
- 1 tbsp. salt
- 1/4 tsp. cardamom

Directions

1. For the ribs, mix all of the marinade ingredients. Marinade the ribs for at least an hour. Mix all of the ingredients for the spice rub.

2. Remove the ribs from the marinade and rub with the spices from the previous step. Heat your grill, and grill for approximately 5 minutes per side. Bon appetite!

Nutritional information (per serving)

Calories: 415
Fat: 32g
Carbs: 1g
Protein: 30g

85. Easy Peezy Pizza

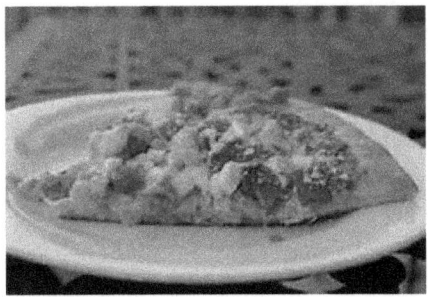

With a crust of mostly egg and cheese, this keto pizza is delicious and customizable with all your favorite toppings!

Serving size: This recipe yields one serving.

Ingredients for the Crust

- 1/2 tsp. Italian seasoning
- 1 tbsp. psyllium husk powder
- Two large eggs
- Two tsp. Frying oil of choice
- 2 tbsp. parmesan cheese
- Salt to taste

Ingredients for the Toppings

- 3 tbsp. tomato sauce
- 1 tbsp. basil (chopped)
- 1.5 oz. mozzarella cheese

Directions

1. Combine all of the pizza crust ingredients. Heat the oil in a frying pan, and add the crust mixture to the pan when hot. Spread into a circle.

2. Once the edges of the crust begin to brown, flip and cook for an additional 60 seconds. Now top the crust with the cheese and

tomato sauce, and broil for 2 minutes until the cheese begins to bubble. Top with basil and enjoy!

Nutritional information (per serving)

Calories: 460
Fat: 36g
Carbs: 4g
Protein: 28g

86. Seared Ribeye

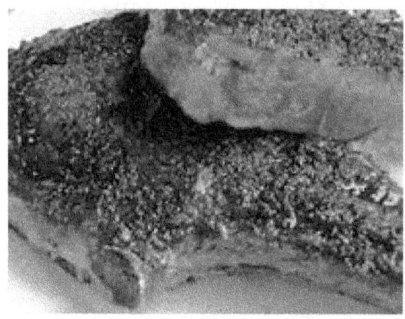

Ribeye, plain and straightforward. Just follow the recipe for searing and combine with your favorite fatty side dishes for a perfect keto friendly dinner!

Serving size: This recipe yields three servings.

Ingredients

- 3 tbsp. bacon fat
- salt and pepper to taste
- Two medium rib eye steaks (about 1.25 lbs.)

Directions

1. Preheat your oven to 250F. Season the steaks with salt and pepper, then place on wire racks for baking. Insert a meat

thermometer into the streak. Bake until the thermometer shows a temperature of 124F.

2. Now heat a cast iron skillet on the stove and add your bacon grease. When scorching, sear your steaks for about 40 seconds per side. All set, eat!

Nutritional information (per serving)

Calories: 425
Fat: 32g
Carbs: 0g
Protein: 31g

87. Keto Salmon and Dill Sauce

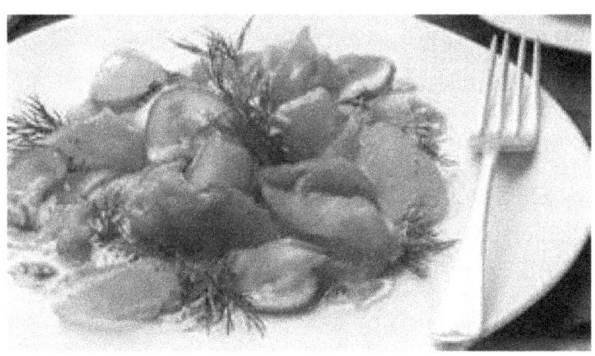

The dill and salmon yields a delectable dish with the full taste of food and a slight tangy hint of dill or sharp mustard. Give this salmon and dill sauce recipe a try and see for yourself!

Serving size: This recipe yields two servings.

Ingredients for the Salmon

- 1 tbsp. duck fat
- One tsp. Tarragon (dried)
- One tsp. Dill weed (dried)

- 1 1/2 lbs. salmon fillet
- Salt and pepper to taste.

Ingredients for the Dill Sauce

- 1/2 tsp. dill weed (dried)
- 1/4 cup heavy cream
- 1/2 tarragon (dried)
- 2 tbsp. butter
- salt and pepper to taste

Directions

1. Slice your salmon, so you have two fillets. Season the meaty side with all of your food spices, and season the skin side with salt and pepper. Heat a skillet over medium, and add the duck fat. When hot, add the salmon with the skin down. Cook for about 5 minutes as the skin crisps.

2. Once the skin is crispy, flip the salmon and reduce heat to low. Cook for about 10 minutes, or until it is cooked to your liking. When the food is removed from the pan, toss in all your spices for the dill sauce, and stir until they begin to turn brown. Add the cream, and stir until hot. Serve it up!

Nutritional information (per serving)

Calories: 465
Fat: 42g
Carbs: 2g
Protein: 23g

88. Orange Duck Breast

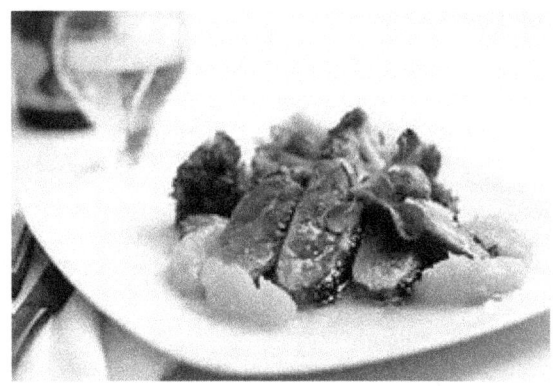

Give your duck some tang by mixing in some orange extract. A fun twist on the traditional duck roast, and sure to be an excellent dinner!

Serving size: This recipe yields one serving.

Ingredients

- 1/2 tsp. orange extract
- 1 tbsp. swerve sweetener
- 1/4 tsp. sage
- 1 tbsp. heavy cream
- 2 tbsp. butter
- 1 cup spinach
- 6 oz. duck breast

Directions

1. Combine all the ingredients. Heat a pan over medium-low, and add the butter and swerve. Cook until the butter begins to brown. Insert the orange extract and sage. Cook until the butter turns dark amber in color.

2. While this is cooking, set another pan on the stove and heat over medium-high. Add the duck breast to this pan. Then flip. Now insert the heavy cream to the butter mixture, and mix well. When hot, pour the mixture over the duck breast and cook for a further

few minutes. Toss the spinach into the pan and cook until wilted. Enjoy!

Nutritional information (per serving)

Calories: 795
Fat: 72g
Carbs: 0g
Protein: 38g

89. Classic Ribeye

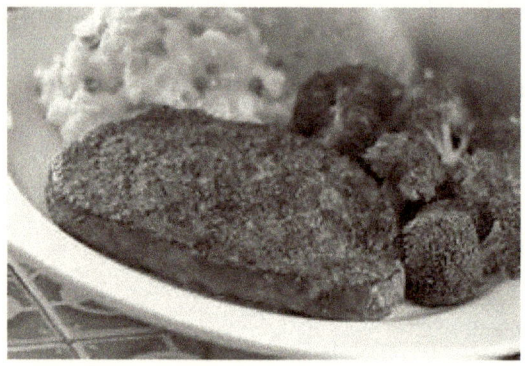

Steak, butter, and duck fat. That's all you need for this delicious ribeye along with some thyme for garnish. Try it with your favorite side dishes and enjoy!

Serving size: This recipe yields two servings.

Ingredients

- One ribeye steak (~16 oz.)
- 1 tbsp. butter
- 1 tbsp. duck fat
- 1/2 tsp. thyme
- Salt and pepper to taste

Directions

1. Preheat your oven to 400F. Place a cast iron skillet in the oven as it is warming. Once the oven is up to temperature, remove the pan and place on the stove over medium heat. Add the oil and steak to the pan. Sear the steak for about 2 minutes.

2. Turn over the steak, and bake in the oven for about 5 minutes. Again, remove the pan, and place over low heat on the stove. Add your butter and thyme to the pan and mix with the oil. Baste the steak for 4 minutes. Let the steak rest for 5 minutes. Put it on your face!

Nutritional information (per serving)

Calories: 748
Fat: 65g
Carbs: 0g
Protein: 39g

90. Chili Turkey Legs

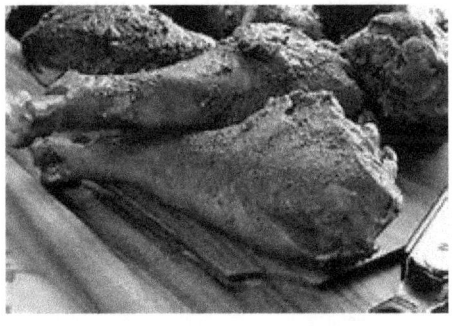

Give those turkey legs some spicy by adding chili powder and cayenne pepper! This recipe is easy to follow and will provide you with a tasty and zippy end to your day.

Serving size: This recipe yields four servings.

Ingredients

- 1/2 tsp. onion powder
- One tsp. Liquid smoke
- 1/2 tsp. thyme (dried)
- 1/2 tsp. pepper
- Two tsp. salt
- 1/4 tsp. cayenne pepper
- 1/2 tsp. garlic powder
- One tsp. Worcestershire sauce
- 1/2 tsp. ancho chili powder
- 2 turkey legs (about 1 lbs. each without bone)
- 2 tbsp. duck fat

Directions

1. Combine all dry spices in a bowl, then toss in the wet ingredients and mix thoroughly. Dry the turkey legs with the paper towel, and then rub in the seasoning. Preheat oven to 350F.

2. Heat a pan over medium-high, and add the duck fat. When the oil begins to smoke, add the turkey legs and sear for 1 to 2 minutes per side. Bake in the oven for 55 to 60 minutes or until thoroughly cooked. That's all folks!

Nutritional information (per serving)

Calories: 380
Fat: 21g
Carbs: 0.5g
Protein: 44g

91. Slow Roasted Pork Shoulder

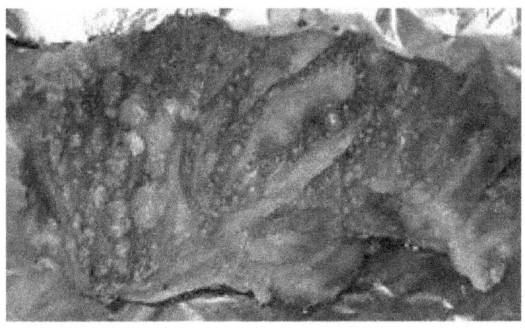

A hearty roasted pork shoulder to round off the day. Simple preparation, keto friendly, and excellent for entertaining!

Serving size: This recipe yields 20 servings.

Ingredients

- One tsp. Black pepper
- Two tsp. oregano
- One tsp. Onion powder
- One tsp. Garlic powder
- 3 1/2 tsp. salt
- 8 lbs. pork shoulder

Directions

1. Preheat oven to 250F. Dry the pork, then rub with the salt and spices. Place the shoulder on a wire rack (a foiled baking sheet works too), and bake for 8 to 10 hours. Remove from the oven, and raise oven temperature to 500F. Cover the shoulder with foil and let rest for about 15 minutes.

2. Remove the foil from the shoulder, and roast in the oven for another 20 minutes, while rotating every 5 minutes. Remove from oven and let rest for 20 minutes. Serve this bad boy up!

Nutritional information (per serving)

Calories: 460
Fat: 35g
Carbs: 0.5g
Protein: 32g

92. Asian Spiced Chicken Thighs

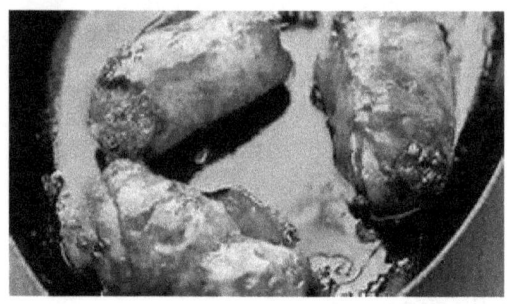

Liven up your chicken thighs with some sriracha and red pepper! These zippy little devils provide an excellent laid-back dinner, or a quick snack during the day!

Serving size: This recipe yields four servings.

Ingredients

- One tsp. Ginger (minced)
- One tsp. Garlic (minced)
- 1/4 tsp. xanthan gum
- 1 tsp. red pepper flakes
- 1 tbsp. ketchup (sugar-free)
- 1 tbsp. olive oil
- 1 tbsp. rice wine vinegar
- Two tsp. sriracha
- 4 cups spinach
- Salt and pepper to taste

Directions

1. Preheat your oven to 425F. Dry your chicken and season the skin with salt and pepper. Mix all of the sauce ingredients until a paste begins to form. Rub this sauce all over the chicken. Lay the chicken on a wire rack

2. Cook the skin is crisp and slight charring appears. Mix the spinach, some salt and pepper, red pepper flakes, and leftover chicken fat together, and serve alongside the baked chicken. Enjoy!

Nutritional information (per serving)

Calories: 600
Fat: 52g
Carbs: 2g
Protein: 30g

93. Baked Poblano Peppers

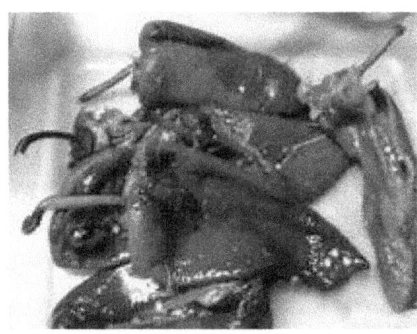

Very similar to baked stuffed mushrooms, these peppers combine pork, mushrooms, cumin, and chili powder for a delicious dinner!

Serving size: This recipe yields four servings.

Ingredients

- Seven baby Bella mushrooms
- 1/2 onion
- 1/4 cup cilantro
- Four poblano peppers
- One tsp. Chili powder
- One tsp. cumin
- 1 tomato
- 1 tbsp. bacon fat
- 1 lb. ground pork
- Salt and pepper to taste

Directions

1. Broil your poblano peppers in the oven for about 10 minutes. Flip or move every couple of minutes to keep boiling consistent. Heat a pan on the stove, and add the bacon fat. Once browned, add the cumin, chili, salt, and pepper. Dice the onion and toss into the mixture, along with the garlic. Fully mix, and then add the mushrooms.

2. Once the mushrooms are cooked, add the cilantro and chopped tomato. Cook for a further 3 minutes. Stuff the poblanos with the mixture and bake at 350F for 9 to 10 minutes. You're all done!

Nutritional information (per serving)

Calories: 365
Fat: 28g
Carbs: 6g
Protein: 22g

94. Coconut Shrimp

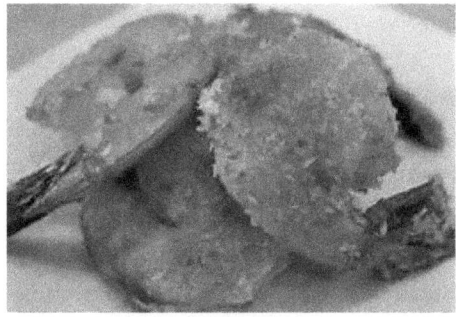

Shrimp with a tropical flair! Coconut crusted with a fruity apricot sauce; this keto recipe will fill you up for dinner and also keep those sweet cravings in check.

Serving size: This recipe yields three servings.

Ingredients for the Shrimp

- 1 cup coconut flakes (unsweetened)
- Two large egg whites
- 1 lb. shrimp (peeled and deveined)
- 2 tbsp. coconut flour

Ingredients for the Sauce

- 1 tbsp. lime juice
- 1 1/2 tbsp. rive wine vinegar
- One medium red chili (diced)
- 1/2 apricot preserves (sugar-free)
- 1/4 tsp. red pepper flakes

Directions

1. Preheat your oven to 400F. Beat the egg whites until soft peaks form. Dip the shrimp in the coconut flour, then dip in the egg whites, then dip in the coconut flakes.

2. Lay the dipped shrimp on a greased baking sheet. Bake the shrimp for 15 minutes. Finish them off with a 3 to 5-minute broil to give them some browning. Mix well. Serve them up and enjoy!

Nutritional information (per serving)

Calories: 395
Fat: 22g
Carbs: 7g
Protein: 37g

95. Slow Cooked Lamb

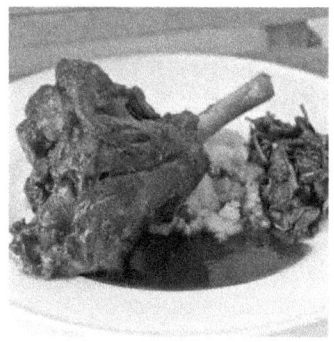

Break out that slow cooker for this affected leg of lamb stuffed with savory herbs. Get it prepared in just a few minutes and let the cooker do the rest!

Serving size: This recipe yields six servings

Ingredients

- 3/4 tsp. rosemary (dried)
- Six leaves mint
- 1 tbsp. maple syrup
- 2 tbsp. whole grain mustard
- 3/4 tsp. garlic
- 1/4 cup olive oil

- 2 lbs. leg of lamb
- Salt and pepper to taste
- 4 sprigs thyme

Directions

1. Slice the lamb. Heat a slow cooker to low, and rub the lamb with olive oil, syrup, mustard, salt, and pepper.

2. Stuff each slit on the lamb with garlic and rosemary. Add to the slow cooker and leave for 7 hours. Add thyme and mint to slow cooker and leave for an additional hour. Enjoy!

Nutritional information (per serving)

Calories: 415
Fat: 35g
Carbs: 0.5g
Protein: 27g

96. Chicken with Paprika

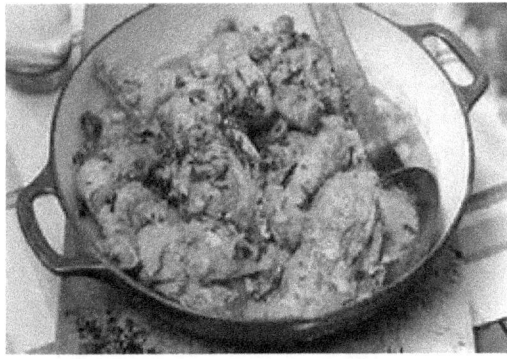

This keto chicken recipe combines sweet and spicy in the form of maple syrup and paprika. Cook this delicious chicken in its sauce then drizzle right before serving.

Serving size: This recipe yields four servings.

Ingredients

- 2 tbsp. Spanish smoked paprika
- 3 tbsp. olive oil
- 1 tbsp. maple syrup
- 2 tbsp. lemon juice
- Two tsp. Garlic (minced)
- Four chicken breasts (boneless and skinless)
- Salt and pepper to taste

Directions

1. Preheat your oven to 350F. Season with the salt and pepper. Combine all other ingredients separately to make the sauce. Add about 1/3 of the sauce to your baking casserole dish or pan. Lay chicken on top of sauce.

2. Drizzle the rest of the sauce over the chicken. Bake for 30 to 35 minutes, and then broil for a further 5 minutes. Serve!

Nutritional information (per serving)

Calories: 275
Fat: 13.5g
Carbs: 2.5g
Protein: 36.5g

97. Curried Chicken Thighs

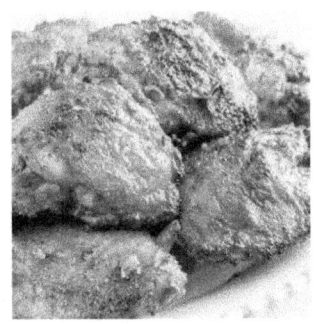

A straight forward, keto friendly method for whipping up some curried chicken. Easy to cook and excellent for those tired weeknights!

Serving size: This recipe yields eight servings.

Ingredients

- 1/2 tsp. chili powder
- 1/2 tsp. coriander (ground)
- 1/2 tsp. cinnamon (ground)
- 1/2 tsp. cayenne pepper
- 1/2 tsp. allspice
- 1/2 tsp. cardamom (ground)
- 1/4 tsp. ginger
- 1 tsp. cumin (ground)
- One tsp. paprika
- 1 tsp. garlic powder
- Two tsp. yellow curry
- Eight chicken thighs (bone in and skin on)
- 1/4 cup olive oil
- 1 1/2 tsp. salt

Directions

1. Preheat oven to 425F. In a bowl, mix all of your spices together. Line a baking sheet with foil, and place all the chicken on the foil.

2. Rub the olive oil and spices over the chicken. Bake for 50 minutes is until thoroughly cooked. Cool for 5 to 8 minutes. Enjoy your evening!

Nutritional information (per serving)

Calories: 278
Fat: 20g
Carbs: 0.5g
Protein: 22g

98. Applewood Pork Chops

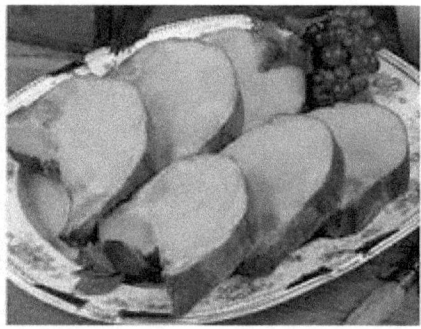

Give your pork chops a subtle hint of Applewood and delicious dinner is all yours! Combine with your favorite fatty side dish, and you have an excellent keto meal right in front of you.

Serving size: This recipe yields four servings.

Ingredients

- 1/2 tsp. garlic powder
- One tsp. Grill Mates Applewood Rub
- 1/2 tsp. black pepper
- 1/2 tsp. Mrs. Dash (table blend)
- 1 tsp. salt
- 2 tbsp. olive oil

- Two 2tsp. Hidden valley powdered ranch
- Four pork chops (bone in)

Directions

1. Combine all of the spices and rub into the pork chops. Heat a pan on medium, and add the olive oil. When hot, add the pork chops and cover. Cook for about 10 minutes and then flip the chops.

2. Cook for a further 5 minutes (covered). Keep the pan uncovered now. Cook for 2 minutes, and then let rest for 4 minutes. Serve and enjoy!

Nutritional information (per serving)

Calories: 260
Fat: 13g
Carbs: 1.5g
Protein: 35g

99. Chicken Stew

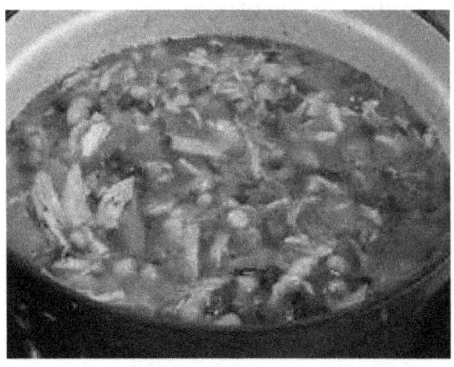

Whether it's a chilly, rainy, or stormy day; good old-fashioned chicken stew is an excellent choice for dinner. Warming and comforting, this recipe fits the bill with some extra zip from hot wing sauce.

Serving size: This recipe yields five servings.

Ingredients

- Two tsp. Garlic (minced)
- 3 tbsp. butter
- Two tsp. paprika
- Two tsp. Ranch seasoning
- One tsp. Red pepper flakes
- One tsp. oregano
- 1/2 cup sliced tomatoes
- One 1/2 tomato sauce
- 3 lbs. chicken thigh
- 1 green pepper
- 1/3 cup hot wing sauce
- 3 cups mushrooms

Directions

1. Finely slice your mushrooms and pepper. Add the legs, tomato slices, garlic, spices, tomato sauce, and hot sauce. Also, toss in peppers and mix. Let the mixture cook for 2 hours.

2. Now turn the pot to low, give the mix a stir, and cook for 4 to 5 hours. Dump in 3 tbsp. Of butter and give another stir. Remove the lid, and cook for an hour. Savor the glory!

Nutritional information (per serving)

Calories: 360
Fat: 22g
Carbs: 8g
Protein: 33g

100. Asian Pork Chops

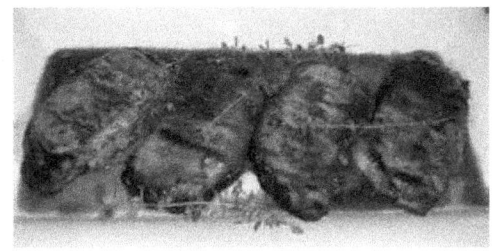

Once again, give the 'old reliable' recipes an upgrade by including some Asian-style spices. Here we have pork chops mixed with anise, soy sauce, and sesame oil to create a unique and enjoyable culinary experience.

Serving size: This recipe yields two servings.

Ingredients

- 1/2 tbsp. sambal chili paste
- 1/2 tsp. five spice
- 1/2 tbsp. ketchup (sugar-free)
- 1 stalk lemon grass
- Four garlic cloves (halved)
- 1 tbsp. almond flour
- 1 tbsp. fish sauce
- 1/2 tsp. peppercorns
- One 1/2 tsp. Soy sauce
- 1 tsp. sesame oil
- 1 medium star anise
- Four boneless pork chops

Directions

1. Pound the pork chops to 1/2-inch thickness. Grind the peppercorns and star anise to a fine powder. Combine the pepper, anise, lemongrass, and garlic. Grind until paste forms. Marinate the chops with the paste. Let the chops marinate for about 2 hours at room temperature.

2. Heat a pan on high. Coat your pork chops with the almond flour. Sear the chops in the pan. It should take about 1 to 2 minutes per side. Once the pork is cooked, cut them into slices. Mix the sambal and ketchup to create your sauce. Enjoy your masterpiece!

Nutritional information (per serving)

Calories: 275
Fat: 10g
Carbs: 5g
Protein: 35g

101. Portobello Burgers

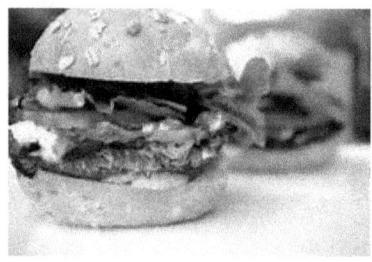

The constant battle to avoid the carbs in bread can be draining. But you can still have a good old-fashioned burger! Dive into this recipe with the twist of mushrooms for the buns.

Serving size: This recipe yields one serving.

Ingredients for the Bun

- 1 tsp. oregano
- 1 clove garlic
- 1/2 tbsp. coconut oil
- 2 Portobello mushroom caps
- 1 pinch each of salt and pepper

Ingredients for the Burger

- One tsp. Each of salt and pepper
- 6 oz. beef
- 1 tbsp. dijon mustard
- 1/4 cup cheddar cheese

Directions

1. Preheat a griddle on high. In a container, combine the oil and spices for the bun. Scrape out the insides of the mushrooms, and marinate in the oil and spices. In a separate bowl, combine the meat, salt, pepper, cheese, and mustard. Use your hands to form your burger patties.

2. Now add your mushrooms to the griddle and cook about 8 minutes. Remove the mushrooms and toss the patties on. Cook about 5 minutes per side. Assemble your burger with whatever toppings you like. That's it!

Nutritional information (per serving)

Calories: 730
Fat: 46g
Carbs: 5g
Protein: 62g

102. BBQ Chicken Pizza

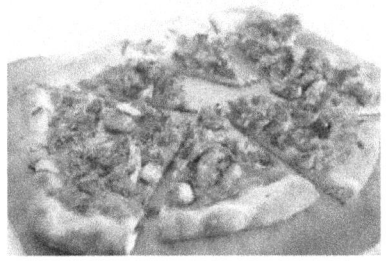

Slash the carbs in your pizza by making your crust out of eggs and cheese! This recipe for BBQ chicken pizza will guide you through the quick and painless process of making your pizza crust, along with some delicious toppings.

Serving size: This recipe yields four servings.

Ingredients for the Crust

- 1 1/2 tsp. Italian seasoning
- 6 tbsp. parmesan cheese
- 3 tbsp. psyllium husk powder
- Six large eggs
- salt and pepper to taste

Ingredients for the Toppings

- 1 tbsp. mayonnaise
- 4 tbsp. tomato sauce
- 6 oz. rotisserie chicken (shredded)
- 4 tbsp. BBQ sauce
- 4 oz. cheddar cheese

Directions

1. Preheat your oven to 425F. Combine all ingredients for the crust in a blender and pulse until thick. An immersion blender will serve this purpose as well.

2. Now spread the dough into a circle on a baking sheet or oven stone. Be sure you grease the surface first. Bake for 10 minutes. Flip the crust over, and pile up your toppings. Boil for a further 10 minutes. Enjoy, you deserve it.

Nutritional information (per serving)

Calories: 355
Fat: 25g
Carbs: 3g
Protein: 25g

103. Cheese Stuffed Burger

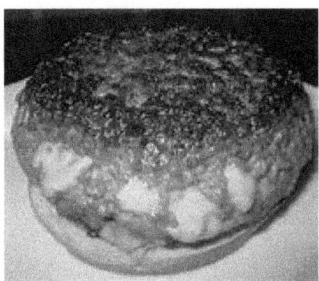

Imagine taking a bit from a juicy burger, and suddenly, there's cheese! The cheese stuffed burger, or the Juicy Lucy, is sure to be a grill or dinnertime favorite.

Serving size: This recipe yields two servings/burgers.

Ingredients

- 1 oz. mozzarella cheese
- 1/2 tsp. pepper
- One tsp salt
- 2 oz. cheddar cheese
- 1 tsp. Cajun seasoning
- 1 tbsp. butter
- Two slices bacon (cooked)
- 8 oz. ground beef

Directions

1. Use your hands to work all the spices into the meat. Form your patties with the mozzarella cheese stuffed inside. Heat a pan on

the stove and add 1 tbsp. Of butter. When hot, add the burger to the pan and cover.

2. Cook 2 to 3 minutes, flip and sprinkle cheese on top. Cover again and cook to taste. Feel fresh to recharge the butter in between burgers if you wish. Chop your bacon and top the burgers. Voila, ready to go!

Nutritional information (per serving)

Calories: 612
Fat: 50g
Carbs: 2g
Protein: 32g

104. Tater Tot Style Nachos

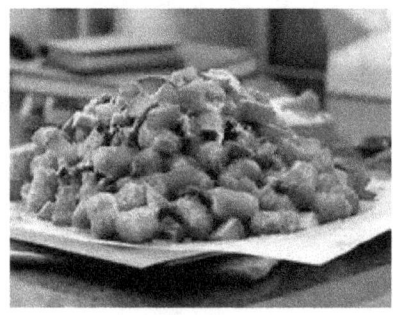

What happens when you combine two cheesy side dishes? You get one amazingly delicious dinner course! This recipe for tater tot nachos tastes just as good as it sounds.

Serving size: This recipe yields two servings.

Ingredients

- Six oz. Ground beef (cooked)
- 2 tbsp. sour cream
- 6 black olives

- 1 tbsp. salsa
- 1/2 jalapeno (sliced)
- 2 oz. cheddar cheese
- Two tater tots (preferably homemade)

Directions

1. In a small cast iron skillet (or casserole dish) place ten children as the base layer. Now add half of your beef and cheddar cheese. Repeat this stack-up again until you use all your ingredients.

2. Broil the dish for about 5 minutes until the cheese is fully melted and bubbly. Serve with the black olives, sour cream, and jalapenos. Enjoy!

Nutritional information (per serving)

Calories: 635
Fat: 53g
Carbs: 6g
Protein: 30g

105. Chipotle Chicken Wings with Blackberry Jam

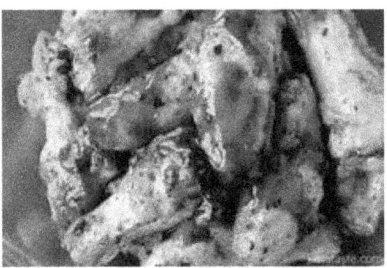

Game day for your favorite team? Have to bring food to a get-together? Then whip up these tasty chipotle style chicken wings! Perfect for sharing or keep them all to yourself, and the blackberry jam in the next recipe makes the perfect side.

Serving size: This recipe yields five servings

Ingredients

- 1/2 cup chipotle jam with blackberries (see next recipe)
- 1/2 cup water
- 3 lbs. chicken wings (~20)
- Salt and pepper to taste

Directions

1. Combine the jam and water in a bowl using a fork or whisk to make sure everything is well mixed. In a plastic bag, add all of the chicken, about 2/3s of the jam, salt, and pepper to taste. Make sure everything is well combined and leave to marinate for at least an hour.

2. Preheat oven to 400F. Bake for 12 minutes. Flip the chicken, crank the temperature to 425F, spread the remaining sauce over the top, and back for another 25 to 30 minutes. Eat as is or add the next recipe in.

Nutritional information (per serving)

Calories: 500
Fat: 40g
Carbs: 1.5g
Protein: 35g

106. Chipotle Jam with Blackberry

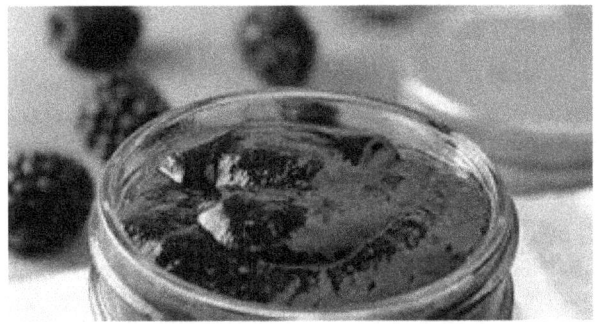

The spicy and fruity combination in this chipotle style blackberry jam makes this sauce an excellent accompaniment to almost any meat. We recommend dishing it up with our recipe for chipotle chicken wings.

Serving size: This recipe yields ten servings/tablespoons.

Ingredients

- 8 drops liquid stevia
- 1/4 cup MCT oil
- 1/4 cup erythritol
- 1/4 tsp. guar gum
- 8 oz. blackberries
- 1 1/2 whole chipotle peppers

Directions

1. Heat a pan over low, and add the blackberries. Cook until they are soft and have released their juices. Add everything except the oil and guar gum to the pan. Use a fork to crush the blackberries and mix well.

2. Now turn up the heat to medium, add the oil, and bring to a boil. Simmer for 8 minutes. Add the guar gum, and mix completely. Stick on the side of a dish or eat solo!

Nutritional information (per serving)

Calories: 50
Fat: 6g
Carbs: 1.5g
Protein: 0.5g

107. Jalapeno Soup

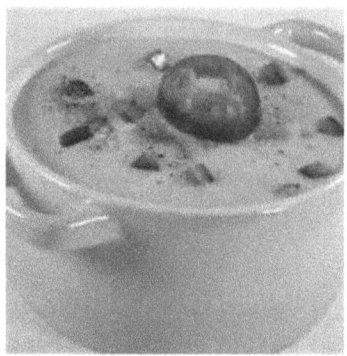

Creamy and full of chicken this recipe will satisfy your spicy side (especially if you keep the jalapeno seeds in!) Serving size:

Serving size: This recipe yields six servings.

Ingredients

- One tsp. Cilantro (dried)
- One tsp. Onion powder
- 1 tsp. Cajun seasoning
- 1 tbsp. chicken fat
- Three jalapenos (diced)
- 3 cups chicken broth
- Four slices bacon (cooked)
- 6 oz. cream cheese
- 4 oz. cheddar cheese
- 4 chicken thighs (deboned)

- salt and pepper to taste
- Two tsp. Garlic (minced)

Directions

1. Preheat your oven to 400F. Rub the seasoning onto the chicken and bake for 50 to 55 minutes. Heat a pan over medium-high and add the chicken fat. Once hot, add your chicken bones and fry them for 10 minutes. Toss in the garlic and jalapenos. Stir and cook for another 4 minutes. Now pour in the broth and spices. Continue to simmer while the chicken bakes.

2. Remove the chicken skin from the thighs and the bones from the pot. Use an immersion blender to puree the jalapenos and garlic. Shred the meat and add to the pan. Simmer for a further 10 minutes. Add the cream cheese and cheddar cheese. Stir to incorporate and simmer for ten more minutes entirely. Garnish with the bacon and enjoy!

Nutritional information (per serving)

Calories: 550
Fat: 43g
Carbs: 4g
Protein: 34g

108. Bacon Cheddar Soup

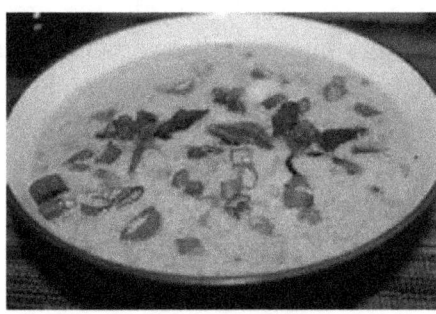

When is it not a good time for bacon and cheese? Yup, that's what we thought. So, dive into this bacon cheddar soup with gusto and enjoy!

Serving size: This recipe yields five servings.

Ingredients

- One tsp. Garlic powder
- 1/2 tsp. celery seed
- 1 tsp. thyme (dried)
- 1 tsp. onion powder
- 3/4 cup heavy cream
- 1/2 tsp. cumin
- 3 cups chicken broth
- Four tbsp. butter
- 1/2 lbs. bacon
- 8 oz. cheddar cheese
- Salt and pepper to taste
- 4 jalapeno peppers (diced)

Directions

1. Chop up the bacon into 1-inch slices. Cook until crisp and save the fat. Now dice your jalapenos and cook in the saved bacon fat. Now toss the bacon fat (we're still using it!) into a pot, along with the butter, spices, and broth. Bring the pot to a boil.

2. Simmer for 15 minutes. Then add the cream and shredded cheese. Stir everything together and keep simmering. Salt and pepper to taste. Add jalapenos and bacon to the pot and simmer for a final 5 minutes. Enjoy!

Nutritional information (per serving)

Calories: 520
Fat: 50g

Carbs: 4g
Protein: 20g

109. Keto Chicken Nuggets

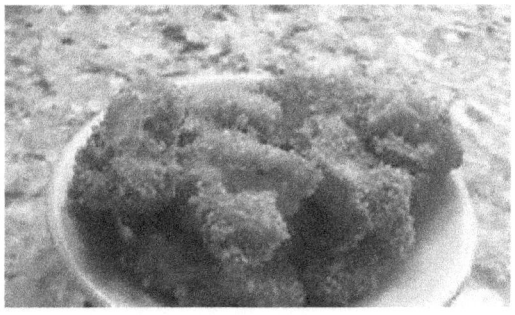

Have a hankering for some fast food chicken nuggets? Then make your keto version! This recipe will satisfy your craving while still keeping you firmly on the ketogenic diet.

Serving size: This recipe yields four servings.

Ingredients for the Nuggets

- 1/4 tsp. paprika
- 1/4 tsp. salt
- 1/4 tsp pepper
- 1/8 tsp. onion powder
- 1/8 tsp. cayenne pepper
- 1/4 tsp. chili powder
- 1/8 tsp. garlic powder
- zest from 1 lime
- 1/4 cup almond flour
- One large egg
- 24 oz. chicken thighs
- 1.5 oz. pork rinds
- 1/4 cup flax meal

Ingredients for the Sauce

- 1 tbsp. lime juice
- 1/8 tsp. cumin
- 1/4 tsp. garlic powder
- 1/2 tsp. red chili flakes
- 1/2 avocado
- 1/2 cup mayonnaise

Directions

1. Mix the ingredients. Put the crumbs in a bowl. Whisk the egg is in the separate container. Lay the chicken on a greased baking tray.

2. Heat the oven to 400F, and back for 15 to 18 minutes. Make the sauce by combining all of the sauce ingredients, and mixing well. Feast!

Nutritional information (per serving)

Calories: 612
Fat: 49g
Carbs: 2g
Protein: 39g

110. Pork Tacos

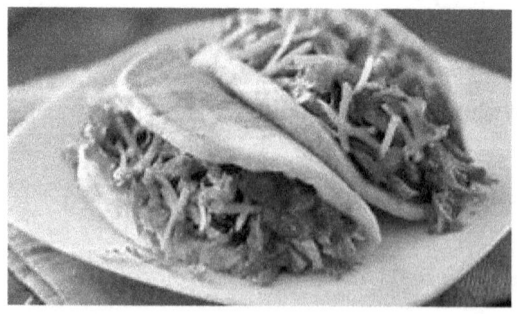

Here's your keto version of the classic pork taco. Pepper, lettuce, and pork and flax seed tortillas; easy to put together and add any other toppings that you feel like!

Serving size: This recipe yields three servings.

Ingredients

- 1/4 tsp. garlic powder
- 1/4 tsp. oregano
- 3/4 yellow pepper
- 1/4 tsp. onion powder
- 1 lbs. pork shoulder (cooked)
- 1 tbsp. olive oil
- 1/2 tsp. salt
- 1/2 tsp. chipotle powder
- One jalapeno pepper
- 1 cup romaine lettuce
- Six thin flax tortillas
- 1/4 tsp. pepper

Directions

1. Chop your pork into cubes. You can also shred it if you wish. Combine all spices and oil, and add to plastic bag. Toss the pork into the plastic bag and marinade for at least 45 minutes. Heat 1 tbsp. Olive oil in a saucepan set over high heat; chop the vegetables and add to pan.

2. When vegetables are done, cook the pork on high heat until completely done and crisp. Assemble your tacos with the vegetables, lettuce, and pork. Enjoy!

Nutritional information (per serving)

Calories: 715

Fat: 68g
Carbs: 3.5g
Protein: 36g

111. Chicken Dressed as Bacon

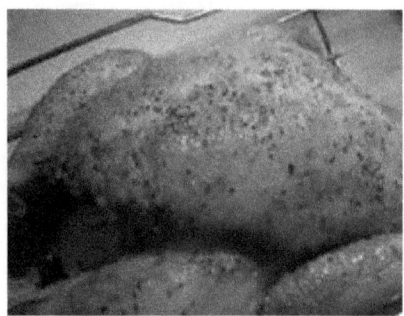

This chick can't pull the wool over our eyes; even though it will look like one giant slab of bacon once you wrap your bacon slices around the outside, and then bake it in a remarkable lemon mustard sauce. Sounds good, doesn't it?

Serving size: This recipe yields eight servings.

Ingredients

- One small lime
- 1 tbsp. grain mustard
- One medium lemon
- Ten strips bacon
- 3 lbs. whole chicken (gutted)
- 4 sprigs fresh thyme
- Salt and pepper to taste

Directions

1. Preheat oven to 500F. Stuff the chicken with the lemon, lime, and thyme. Season bacon with salt and pepper and wrap over the

chicken any way you wish. Add the chicken to a roasting pan, and bake for 15 minutes.

2. Lower temperature to 350F, and bake for a further 45 minutes. Transfer the fat and juice to a stovetop pan. Bring the pan to a boil and add mustard. Mix well. Serve with the sauce on the side!

Nutritional information (per serving)

Calories: 375
Fat: 30g
Carbs: 2g
Protein: 24g

112. Keto Fried Chicken

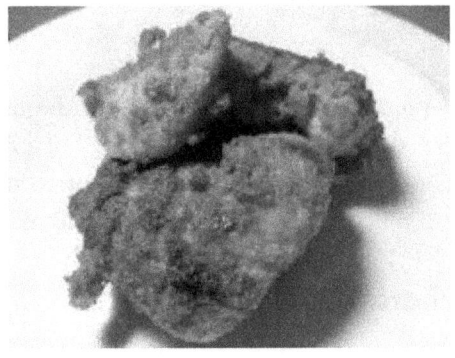

Serving size: This recipe yields 10 servings.

Ingredients

- Ten pieces of Chicken
- 3/4 cup of Plain Whey Protein
- One cup of Crushed Pork Rinds
- 1/2 teaspoon of Onion Powder
- 1 tablespoon of Oat Fiber
- 1/2 cup of Parmesan Cheese

- 2 Large Eggs
- 1/4 cup of Heavy Cream
- 1/4 cup of Water
- 3/4 inch of Deep Hot Oil
- 1/8 teaspoon of Coarse Black Pepper

Directions

1. Measure out and then mix all your dry ingredients in a paper bag. Shake it well. Whisk eggs, water, and cream together in your large-sized bowl. Toss in your pieces of cut up chicken into your egg mix and coat each piece thoroughly.

2. Take pieces out of your bowl and drop in your bag of seasoned flour. When three parts are in your bag, hold the top closed and shake your bag to coat chicken. Heat 3/4-inch cheap oil on a high heat.

3. Place your pieces close together. Lower the heat to a medium-high. Brown your chicken on one side. Turn over carefully and brown the opposite side. Should take approximately 30 minutes. Remove and place on your paper towel. Serve!

113. Keto Chicken Divan

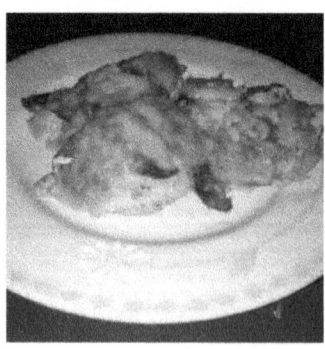

Serving size: This recipe yields 6 servings.

Ingredients

- 2 Boneless Chicken Breasts
- Three tablespoons of Ghee
- 1 Small Yellow Onion
- 3 cups of Steamed Chopped Broccoli
- 1/2 Tablespoon of Minced Garlic
- 1 cup of Chicken Stock or Broth
- 3 cups of Cauliflower
- One teaspoon of Lemon Juice
- 1/2 cup of Mayonnaise
- 1 cup of Heavy Cream
- 2 cups of Shredded Cheddar Cheese
- Ten cranks of Fresh Pepper
- 1/2 teaspoon of Garlic Salt
- Dash of Parsley

Directions

1. Preheat your oven to 350 degrees. Fill your pot halfway with water. Add in your chicken breasts. Boil until your chicken is cooked. Cook your onions and garlic in a medium frying pan over a low heat with your ghee.

2. While that cook, blend your cauliflower using your food processor. Do this for a few seconds until it looks like rice. After cooking your onions for 2 minutes, add in your spices one by one mixing each one in.

3. Once your onions are nice and soft, add in your cauliflower. Once your cauliflower gets soft, add in your chicken broth. Cover and cook for approximately 10 minutes. Take out your chicken once it's done.

4. Add your lemon juice and cream. Allow it to simmer uncovered over a low heat for approximately 10 minutes. Mix a few times,

so your bottom doesn't burn. Add in your mayo and mix. Turn off your burner.

5. Pull your chicken apart. Add in half of your pulled chicken into cauliflower cream mix. Use other 1/2 to line your 8x8-inch casserole dish. On top of your bottom chicken layer, place your steamed chopped broccoli. Top with your cauliflower cream mix.

6. Top that with your cheddar cheese. Place in oven for approximately 30 minutes. Cover it with tinfoil. Remove your paper and cook for about 10 minutes. Serve!

114. Bolognese Zoodle Bake

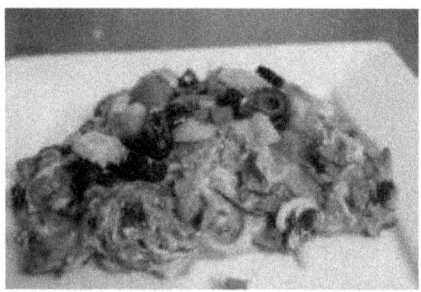

Serving size: This recipe yields 6 servings.

Ingredients for the Bolognese Sauce

- 1 1/2 pounds of Ground Beef
- 1/2 Medium White Onion
- One tablespoon of Olive Oil
- 2 cups of Rao's Marinara Sauce
- Three Cloves of Minced Garlic
- 1/2 teaspoon of Thyme
- 1/4 cup of Chicken Bouillon Paste
- 1/2 teaspoon of Ground Marjoram
- 1/2 teaspoon of Ground Nutmeg
- Two tablespoons of Heavy Whipping Cream

- Salt
- Pepper

Ingredients for the Zucchini Noodles

- 3 Medium Zucchini
- Two tablespoons of Olive Oil
- 1 cup of Shredded Mozzarella Cheese
- Salt
- Pepper
- Fresh Basil (Optional)

Directions

1. Set your slow cooker on "low." Finely dice half of your medium-sized white onion while you wait for your skillet to heat up. Add your olive oil to your frying pan. Once your oil becomes hot, add your diced onion. Stir in your minced garlic cloves.

2. Crumble your ground beef into the pan. Don't worry too much about breaking up the chunks as they cook. Everything is going to fall apart in the slow cooker anyway. Add in 1/2 a teaspoon of thyme, 1/2 a teaspoon of nutmeg, 1/2 a teaspoon of marjoram, and black pepper.

3. Mix everything together and allow your beef to cook until it has mostly browned. Stir in 2 tablespoons of your heavy whipping cream. Finish the sauce by mixing in 1/4 of a cup of your chicken bouillon. Be careful not to pour hot sauce into cold stoneware.

4. Cover your slow cooker and allow your sauce to simmer for about 8 hours. Stir occasionally to prevent burning. Preheat your oven to 350 degrees. Set up a vegetable spiralizer. Use it to process the zucchini into noodles, and place the noodles in a casserole dish. Break apart the longer strands so that none of them are too long.

5. Add two tablespoons of olive oil to your noodles. Season to taste and then mix. Spread your Bolognese sauce over the top of your zucchini. Top your casserole with 1 cup of shredded mozzarella cheese.

6. If baking right after cooking the Bolognese sauce, then you will only need to heat the pan in the oven for approximately 15 to 20 minutes. If you've made the sauce ahead of time and it's been chilled in the refrigerator, then you will need to bake for 30 to 35 minutes. Garnish with fresh basil if desired. Serve!

Nutritional Value

402 Calories.
29 grams of Protein.
6 grams of Carbs.
29 grams of Fat.

115. Skillet Browned Chicken w/ Creamy Greens

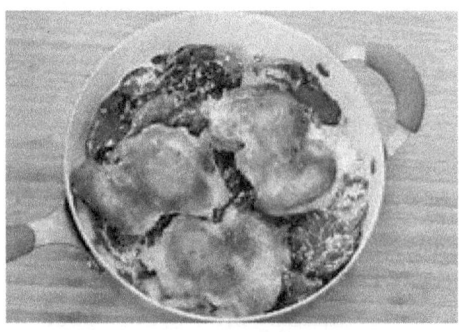

Serving size: This recipe yields 4 servings.

Ingredients

- 1 pound of Boneless Chicken Thighs
- 1 cup of Chicken Stock
- Two tablespoons of Coconut Oil

- 2 Tablespoons of Melted Butter
- 1 cup of Cream
- One teaspoon of Italian Herbs
- 2 tablespoons of Coconut Flour
- 2 cups of Dark Leafy Greens
- Pepper
- Salt

Directions

1. Preheat your large-sized skillet on a medium-high setting. Add two tablespoons of coconut oil to your pan. Season both sides of your chicken thighs with salt and pepper while your oil heats up. Brown your chicken thighs in the skillet. Fry both sides until your chicken is cooked through and crispy. While your legs are cooking, you should start the sauce.

2. To create your sauce, melt two tablespoons of butter in your saucepan. Once your butter stops sizzling, whisk in 2 tablespoons of coconut flour to form a thick paste. Whisk in 1 cup of cream and bring to a boil.

3. Remove your cooked chicken thighs from the skillet and set to the side. Pour the cup of chicken stock into your chicken skillet and deglaze the pan. Whisk in your cream sauce. Stir the greens into your pan so that they become coated with your sauce. Lay your chicken thighs back on top of the greens, then remove from the heat and serve. Divide your chicken and greens up into four servings. Serve!

Nutritional Value

446 Calories.
18 grams of Protein.
2 grams of Carbs.
38 grams of Fat.

116. BBQ Bacon Cheeseburger Waffles

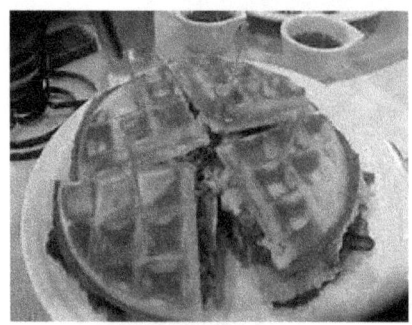

Serving size: This recipe yields 4 servings.

Ingredients for the Waffles

- 1 1/2 ounces of Cheddar Cheese
- 3 tablespoons of Parmesan Cheese
- 2 Large Eggs
- Four tablespoons of Almond Flour
- 1 cup of Cauliflower Crumbles
- Pepper

Ingredients for the Topping

- 4 ounces of Ground Beef (70/30)
- 4 slices of Chopped Bacon
- Four tablespoons of Sugar-Free BBQ Sauce
- 1 1/2 ounces of Cheddar Cheese Salt
- Pepper

Directions

1. Shred up 3 ounces worth of cheese. Half will go into your waffle, and half will go on top, so make sure you keep it to the side. Mix in half of your cheddar cheese, Parmesan cheese, eggs, almond flour, and spices. Set to the side. Slice your bacon thin and cook

over medium-high heat. Once your bacon is partially cooked, add in your beef. Add any excess grease from your pan into your waffle mixture that you have set to the side. Immersion blend your waffle mixture into a thick paste.

2. Add half of your mixture to your waffle iron and cook until it's crisp. Keep in mind that cauliflower waffles tend to take a little bit longer to cook (there's much more moisture). A good rule of thumb to use is that the waffle is finished once there is little to no steam coming from the waffle iron. Repeat for the second waffle.

3. While your waffles are cooking, add in your sugar-free BBQ sauce to the bacon and ground beef mixture in your pan. Assemble your waffles together by adding half of the ground beef mixture and half of the remaining cheddar cheese to the top of your waffle. Boil until your cheese is nicely melted over the top. Slice up your green onion while your pizzas are broiling to sprinkle over the top. Serve!

Nutritional Value

354 Calories.
19 grams of Protein.
3 grams of Carbs.
30 grams of Fat.

117. Chicken Thighs w/ Spinach

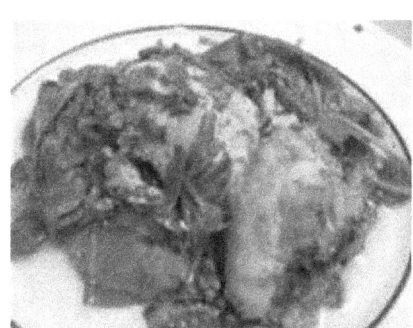

Serving size: This recipe yields 8 servings.

Ingredients

- 16 Boneless Chicken Thighs (Skinless)
- 2 tablespoons of Shredded Cheddar Cheese
- 24 ounces of Spinach
- 2 cups of Water
- Garlic
- Salt
- Pepper

Directions

1. Place your chicken thighs into your roaster pan covered with your lid. Bake at 350 degrees for approximately 2 hours. Remove and allow it to cool. Place two thighs each in 8 different containers.

2. Break up your legs and put your vegetables and cheese on each. Distribute your leftover juices over the chicken in each bowl. Serve!

Nutritional Value

390 Calories.
45 grams of Protein.
3 grams of Carbs.
23 grams of Fat.

118. Loaded Baked Chicken

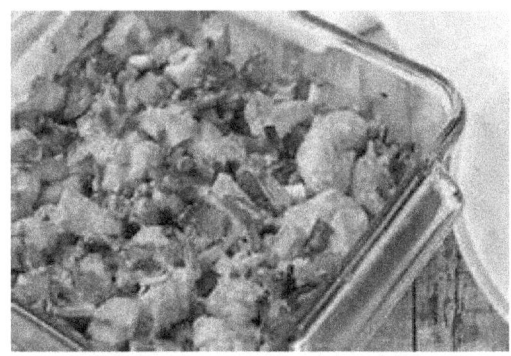

Serving size: This recipe yields 4 servings.

Ingredients

- 4 Chicken Breasts
- 4 Bacon Strips
- 1 ounce of Soy Sauce
- 3 Green Onions

Directions

1. Heat your cast iron pan and cook your oil on a high heat. Pan fry your chicken breasts. Flip them half way through. Total cook time should be approximately 10 to 15 minutes. Internal temperature should be 165 degrees.

2. While your chicken cooks, cook your bacon and crumble into bits when done. Chop up your green onions. Place your chicken in your baking dish. Top it with your soy sauce, then add your ranch, bacon, green onions, and your cheese. Broil on high for approximately 3 to 4 minutes until your cheese melts. Serve!

Nutritional Value

527 Calories.
63 grams of Protein.
3 grams of Carbs.

28 grams of Fat.

119. Beer Can Chicken

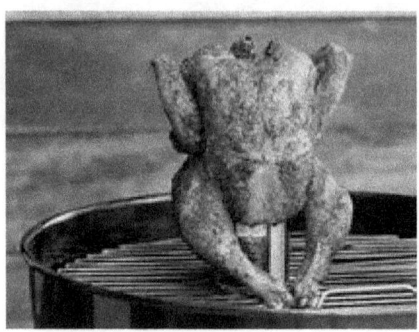

Serving size: This recipe yields 4 servings.

Ingredients

- One Whole Chicken
- One tablespoon of Bacon Fat
- 1 can of Beer
- Rotisserie Seasoning

Directions

1. Preheat your grill to medium-high heat, Set it up for indirect grilling. No heat under the chicken. Remove and get rid of your gizzards from your thawed chicken. Cut away the loose skin and chicken parts from the opening of breast cavity. Dry it on both the outside and inside.

2. Apply oil or bacon fat to the outside of your chicken. Rub in your Rotisserie seasoning on both inside and outside. Remove half of the beer from the can and set your chicken on the can. Grill for approximately 60 minutes or until your meat reads between 165 and 180 degrees. Serve!

120. Garlic Lebanese Chicken Thighs

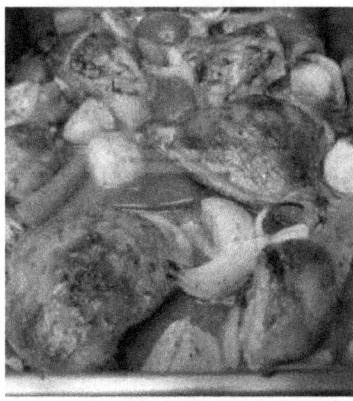

Serving size: This recipe yields 2 servings.

Ingredients

- 4 Chicken Thighs
- 1 Vidalia Onion (Quartered)
- 2 Roma Tomatoes
- 2 tablespoons of Ghee
- 15 whole cloves of Garlic
- 1 Juiced Fresh Lemon
- Handful of Baby Carrots
- Garlic Olive Oil
- Oregano
- Pepper
- Salt

Directions

1. Heat your oven to 500 degrees. Glaze the bottom of your cast iron pan with 2 teaspoons of garlic olive oil. Add your four chicken thighs together. Make sure some space separates them. Wedge your carrots, onions, tomatoes, and garlic cloves between your chicken legs. Add two garlic cloves on top of the thighs. Juice

your lemon over your chicken thighs. Put garlic the on top of your chicken thighs. Drizzle ghee over your chicken thighs.

2. Sprinkle your oregano over your dish. Add your pepper and salt. Place in oven for approximately 30 minutes. Reduce your heat to 350 degrees and then cook about 20 minutes until cooked to an internal temperature of 165 degrees. Place your oven on broil and cook an additional 5 minutes until outside the skin is crispy. Remove from your oven. Serve!

121. Tequila Chicken

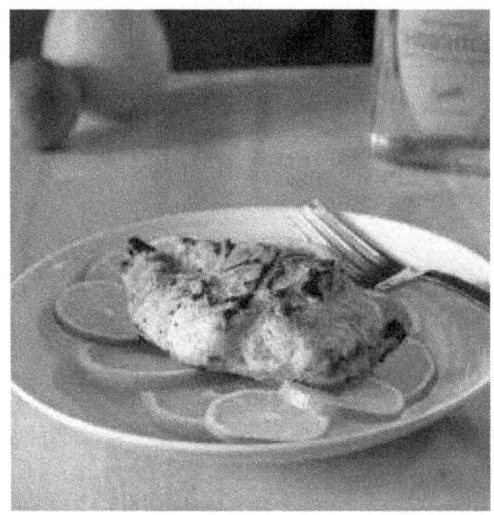

Serving size: This recipe yields 6 servings.

Ingredients for the Marinade

- 6 Chicken Breasts
- 1/2 teaspoon of Garlic Powder
- 1 cup of Water
- 1/2 teaspoon of Liquid Smoke
- 1/4 cup of Soy Sauce
- Two tablespoons of Lime Juice

- One shot of Tequila (50 ml)
- 1/2 teaspoon of Salt

Ingredients for the Sauce

- 1/4 cup of Sour Cream
- 1/4 cup of Tomato Sauce
- 1/4 cup of Mayonnaise
- 1/4 teaspoon of Frank's Hot Sauce
- One tablespoon of Heavy Cream
- Pepper 1/4 teaspoon of Dried Parsley
- 6 ounces of Shredded Cheddar Cheese
- 1/4 teaspoon of Paprika
- Ground Cumin 1/4 teaspoon of Salt
- 1/4 teaspoon of Black Pepper

Directions

1. Mix your marinade ingredients. Add your chicken to the marinade. Allow it to sit and refrigerate for approximately 2 to 3 hours. Place your chicken on your broiler pan and then broil for about 20 minutes on high. Flip it after 10 minutes. Check chicken for temperature. You want it to get to 165 degrees internally.

2. Mix all your ingredients for your sauce except the cheese. Place your meat in your casserole dish. Cover it with sauce and your cheese. Broil for three more minutes on high. Cheese should be a little bubbly. Serve!

Nutritional Value

445 Calories.
60 grams of Protein.
2 grams of Carbs.
22 grams of Fat.

122. Pounded Chicken Pizza

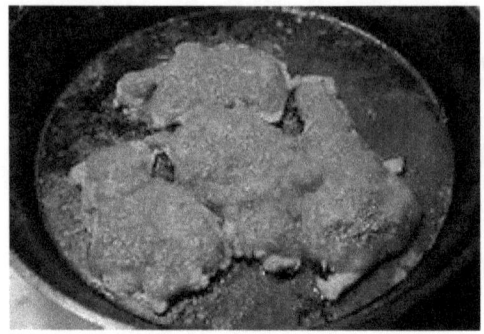

Serving size: This recipe yields 4 servings.

Ingredients

- Four Chicken Thighs
- 16 slices of Pepperoni
- 2 1/2 ounces of Shredded Jarlsberg Cheese
- 4 slices of Bacon
- 2 1/2 ounces of Shredded Cheddar Cheese
- 1/2 cup of Marinara Sauce
- 1 ounce of Shredded Monterey Cheese
- Italian Seasoning
- Pepper
- Salt

Directions

1. Preheat your oven to 350 degrees. Start cooking your four slices of bacon. Place your chicken thighs on cutting board. Cover it with saran wrap. Pound it with your heavy pan. Pepper and salt both sides of your chicken. Heat up grease in your pan over high heat. Sear your chicken on each side for 1 minute.

2. Transfer your skillet to your oven and cook for approximately 10 minutes. Remove your skillet from the oven. Add your seasoning

and sauce. Cover it with cheese and place back in your oven for approximately 3 minutes on broil. Remove from oven. Add your remaining toppings. It includes pepperoni and bacon. Cook for two more minutes. Serve!

Nutritional Value

461 Calories.
32 grams of Protein.
1 gram of Carbs.
36 grams of Fat.

123. Beer Can Burgers

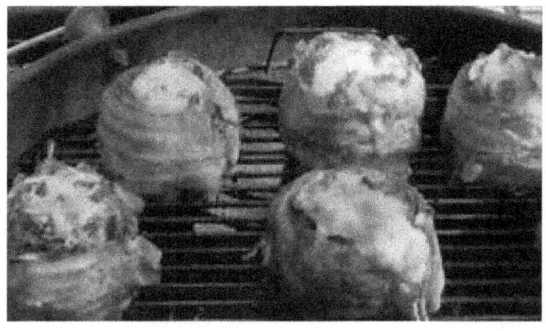

Serving size: This recipe yields 5 servings.

Ingredients

- 50 ounces of Ground Beef
- 2 1/2 ounces of Pepper Jack Cheese (Cubed)
- Ten slices of Bacon
- 2 1/2 ounces of Shredded Extra Sharp Cheddar Cheese
- 6 ounces of Cooked Sliced Fresh Mushrooms
- 6 ounces of Cooked Brussels Sprouts
- 6 ounces of Cooked Green Peppers
- 6 ounces of Cooked Onions

Directions

1. Preheat your grill to 300 degrees. Set it up for indirect heat. Divide your ground beef into equal amounts and make them into giant balls. Push a can into your ball and smush it. Using your hand, form the meat around your can, making sure to push it up evenly around your can. Wrap 2 pieces of bacon around the base of your meat.

2. Extract your can and fill the hole with whatever you'd like. In this example, we used green peppers, onions, brussels sprouts, and mushrooms. Top it with your cheese. Place on your grill and cook over indirect heat for approximately 1 hour. Take off your grill. Serve!

Nutritional Value

963 Calories.
66 grams of Protein.
8 grams of Carbs.
73 grams of Fat.

Keto Snacks

124. Keto 5 Layer Dip

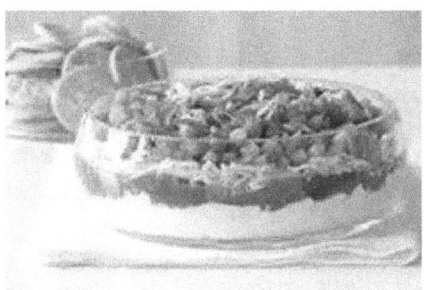

Serving size: This recipe yields 10 servings.

Ingredients

- 20 ounces of Guacamole
- 4 ounces of Diced Green Onions
- 8 ounces of Sour Cream
- 4 ounces of Mayo
- 16 ounces of Salsa
- 4 ounces of Cream Cheese
- 10 ounces of Shredded Cheddar Cheese
- Two tablespoons of Taco Seasoning

Directions

1. Combine your mayo, cream cheese, sour cream, and seasoning. Mix until smooth. Chop your green onions. Layer 1 - Use your medium-sized casserole dish and spread out your guacamole on the bottom.

2. Tier 2 - Carefully spread your sour cream mix over the top your guacamole. Layer 3 - Spread your salsa over your sour cream mixture.

3. Layer 4 - Add your cheese. Tier 5 - Top with your green onions. Refrigerate it for at least 1 hour. Serve!

Nutritional Value

343 Calories.
10 grams of Protein.
11 grams of Carbs.
29 grams of Fat.

125. Spicy Bacon Cauliflower

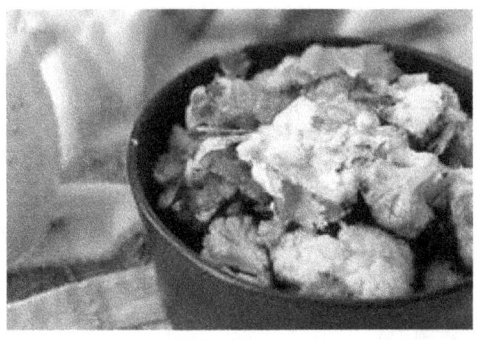

Serving size: This recipe yields 4 servings.

Ingredients

- 16 ounces of Frozen Cauliflower
- Five slices of Thick Cut Bacon
- Old Bay

Directions

1. Microwave your entire bag of cauliflower. Cook your bacon until it is crisp in your oven at 450 degrees. Heat your bacon grease in your skillet. Add your cooked cauliflower to your fat and cover slowly with your Old Bay.

2. Saute this for approximately 5 minutes. Be sure to mix around well. Reapply your Old Bay. Mix until your cauliflower is well cooked and broken up. Take your bacon out of your oven and cut into small pieces. Add it to your mixture. Serve!

Nutritional Value

100 Calories.
6 grams of Protein.
5 grams of Carbs.
6 grams of Fat.

126. Cheesy Cauliflower Onion Dip

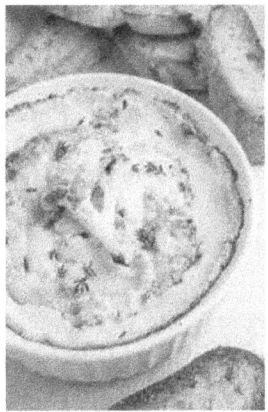

Serving size: This recipe yields 24 servings.

Ingredients

- 1 pound of Cauliflower
- 1/2 cup of Onion
- 1 1/2 cups of Chicken Broth
- 3/4 cup of Cream Cheese
- 1/4 cup of Mayonnaise
- 1/2 teaspoon of Ground Cumin
- 1/2 teaspoon of Garlic Powder

- 1/2 teaspoon of Chili Powder
- 1/2 teaspoon of Ground Black Pepper
- 1/2 teaspoon of Salt

Directions

1. Simmer your cauliflower and onion in your chicken broth until soft and tender. Stir in your garlic powder, cumin, chili powder, pepper, and salt. Cut up chunks of your cream cheese and whisk into your cauliflower until the cream cheese melts and is no longer chunky.

2. Use a blender to blend your mixture until it's smooth. Carefully whisk in your mayonnaise. Chill in your fridge for approximately 2 to 3 hours. Serve!

Nutritional Value

51 Calories.
1 grams of Protein.
1 grams of Carbs.
4 grams of Fat.

127. Pesto Keto Crackers

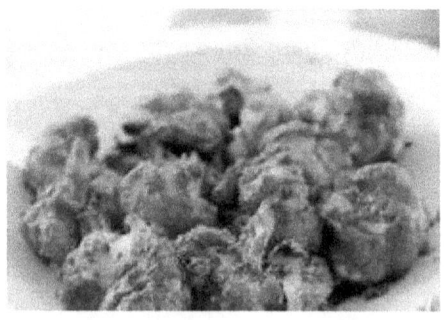

Serving size: This recipe yields 6 servings.

Ingredients

- 1 1/4 cups of Almond Flour
- 1/4 teaspoon of Dried Basil
- 1/2 teaspoon of Baking Powder
- 1 clove of Pressed Garlic
- Three tablespoons of Butter
- Two tablespoons of Basil Pesto
- Pinch of Cayenne Pepper
- 1/4 teaspoon of Ground Black Pepper
- 1/2 teaspoon of Salt

Directions

1. Preheat your oven to 325 degrees. Line your cookie sheet with parchment paper. In your medium-sized bowl, combine your almond flour, pepper, salt and baking powder and whisk until smooth. Add your basil, cayenne, and garlic and stir until evenly combined. Add in your pesto and whisk until your dough forms into coarse crumbs.

2. Cut the butter into your cracker mixture with a fork or your fingers until your dough forms into a ball. Transfer your dough onto the prepared cookie sheet and spread out your dough thinly until it's about 1 1/2 mm thick. Make sure the thickness is the same throughout so that the crackers bake evenly.

3. Place your pan in the preheated oven and bake for approximately 14 to 17 minutes until light golden brown in color. Once your dough has finished cooking, remove it from the oven. Cut into crackers of your desired size or allow it to cool and then break it into pieces. Serve!

Nutritional Value

210 Calories.

5 grams of Protein.
3 grams of Carbs.
20 grams of Fat.

128. Mini Pumpkin Spice Muffins

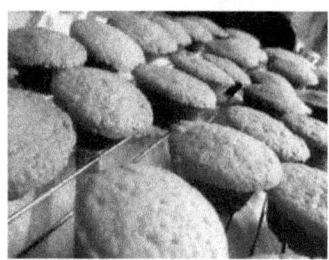

Serving size: This recipe yields 18 servings.

Ingredients

- 3/4 cup of Canned Pumpkin
- 1 Large Egg (Room Temperature)
- 1/4 cup of Organic No Sugar Added Sunflower Seed Butter
- 1/2 teaspoon of Ground Nutmeg
- 1/2 cup of Erythritol
- Two tablespoons of Organic Flaxseed Meal
- 1/4 cup of Organic Coconut Flour (Sifted)
- 1/2 teaspoon of Baking Powder
- One teaspoon of Ground Cinnamon
- Three tablespoons of Plain Cream Cheese (Optional)

Directions

1. Preheat your oven to 350 degrees then lightly grease your mini muffin pan. You will need 18 sections to bake your entire recipe. Then in your mixing bowl combine your pumpkin, sunflower seed butter, and your egg. Stir until smooth. Add all of your remaining dry ingredients.

2. Stir to blend. Using a 1-tablespoon measuring spoon, scoop your batter into your prepared pan. Bake approximately 15 minutes, then remove your pan from the oven and allow it to cool completely.

3. Carefully take off your muffins from your pan and transfer to your serving tray. You can optionally top your cupcakes with cream cheese. You may also refrigerate your muffins up to 1 week, or freeze up to 1 month. They are best when warmed slightly if refrigerated or frozen. If freezing, do not top with cream cheese until thawed. Serve!

Nutritional Value

43 Calories.
2 grams of Protein.
2.5 grams of Carbs.
3 grams of Fat.

129. Keto Tortilla Chips

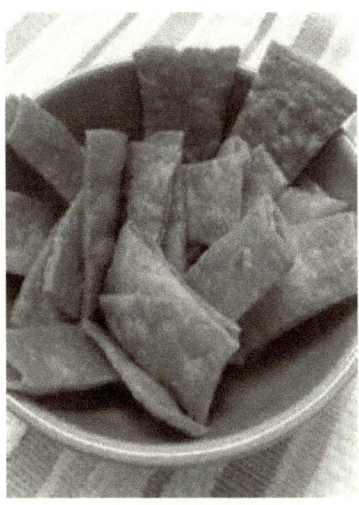

Serving size: This recipe yields 36 servings.

Ingredients for the Tortilla Chips

- 6 Tortillas
- Three tablespoons of Oil
- Pepper
- Salt

Ingredients for the Optional Toppings

- Diced Jalapeno
- Shredded Cheese
- Fresh Salsa
- Full-Fat Sour Cream

Directions

1. Cut your tortillas into chip-sized slices. I got 6 out of each tortilla. Heat your deep fryer. Once ready, lay out the pieces of your tortilla in your basket. You can fry 4 to 6 pieces at a time.

2. Fry for about 1 to 2 minutes, then flip. Continue to cook for another 1 to 2 minutes on the other side. Remove from your fryer and place on paper towels to cool. Add your toppings of choice. Serve!

Nutritional Value

27 Calories.
1 gram of Protein.
.04 grams of Carbs.
3 grams of Fat.

130. Bacon Brussels Sprouts

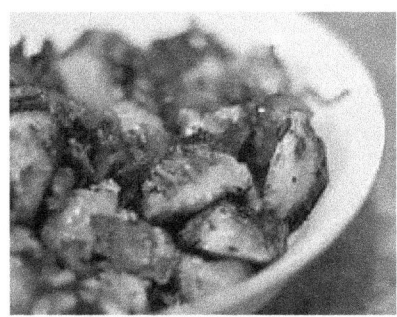

Serving size: This recipe yields 4 servings.

Ingredients

- 1/4 cup of Fish Sauce
- Six strips of Bacon
- 24 ounces of Brussels Sprouts
- Pepper

Directions

1. De-stem and quarter your brussels sprouts. Mix your brussels sprouts, fish sauce, and bacon grease. Cook your bacon. Once done cut into smaller strips. Add your bacon to your mix and add some pepper. Stir together well. On your greased pan spread out your brussels sprouts.

2. Cook for approximately 40 minutes at 450 degrees, stirring in 10-minute intervals. Finish off your brussels sprouts on broil for a couple of minutes. Serve!

Nutritional Value

143 Calories.
6 grams of Protein.
8 grams of Carbs.
10 grams of Fat.

131. Kohlrabi Kraut

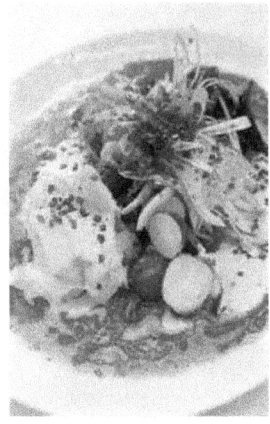

Serving size: This recipe yields 12 servings.

Ingredients

- 2 pounds of Ham Hock
- 12 ounces of Salt Pork
- 4 Shredded Kohlrabi
- 1/2 of an Onion
- 1/2 cup of Champagne Vinegar
- 1 teaspoon of Caraway Seeds

Directions

1. Fill your large-sized pot halfway with water and boil on a high heat. Add your bacon grease to your skillet and heat on high. Cut up 1/4 of an onion.

2. Brown your ham hocks in bacon fat. Add your onions to your pan and fry with your ham hocks. Once your onions get cooked, and ham hocks are browned, add to boiling water and season with your pepper and salt.

3. Peel and quarter your kohlrabi. Grate your kohlrabi in your food processor. Grate 1/4 of an onion into your mix. Add your kohlrabi to water and season it with your pepper and salt.

4. Add your caraway seeds and champagne vinegar. Cover and allow it to simmer approximately 3 hours. Stir occasionally. If water gets low while simmering add more. The mixture should be covered with water for entire 3 hours. Near the end of simmer remove ham hocks and separate the bone from the meat. Add your meat back into your pot. Serve!

Nutritional Value

181 Calories.
14 grams of Protein.
7 grams of Carbs.
17 grams of Fat.

132. Bacon Rollups

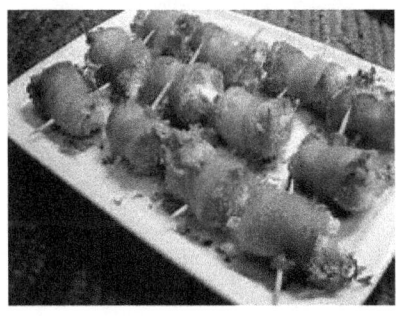

Serving size: This recipe yields 1 serving.

Ingredients

- Two slices of Bacon
- Two slices of Cheddar Cheese
- 2 Toothpicks

Directions

1. Cut each cheese piece vertically into fours. Cook your bacon until it is crisp. Remove your bacon and add your cheese quickly. Roll up and skewer your roll. Let your bacon crisp and allow your cheese to melt a little bit. Serve!

Nutritional Value

135 Calories.
9 grams of Protein.
0 grams of Carbs.
12 grams of Fat.

133. Cheddar Garlic Biscuits

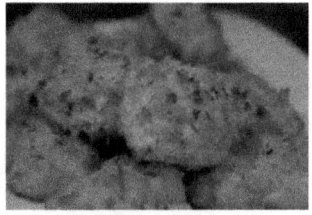

Serving size: This recipe yields 37 serving.

Ingredients

- 6 ounces of Shredded Colby Jack Cheese
- 2 Large Eggs
- Two teaspoons of Granulated Garlic
- 2 1/2 cups of Almond Flour
- 8 ounces of Cream Cheese
- Five tablespoons of Butter
- 3/4 teaspoon of Xanthan Gum
- One teaspoon of Baking Soda
- 1 teaspoon of Sea Salt

Directions

1. Line your cookie sheet with some parchment paper. In your food processor place your shredded cheese and 1 cup of almond flour. Process until finely grained. Put to the side. In your glass mixing bowl, place your cream cheese and butter. Microwave for 30 seconds. Whisk until glossy and smooth.

2. Whisk in your eggs until it is smooth. Mix in your baking soda, garlic, salt, and xanthan gum. Add your almond flour cheese mix to egg mixture. Add your remaining almond flour and fold in until it is mixed well and a dough begins forming.

3. Drop dough by tablespoon onto your cookie sheet. Space each an inch apart. Roll dough a bit to smooth it out, so it makes a prettier biscuit. Bake approximately 20 to 25 minutes. Should be golden brown on top. Remove and allow it to cool down for 10 minutes. Serve!

Nutritional Value

96 Calories.
3 grams of Protein.
Two grams of Carbs.
9 grams of Fat.

134. Turnip Hash Browns

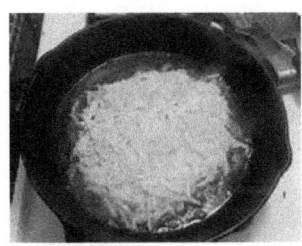

Serving size: This recipe yields 2 servings.

Ingredients

- 1 Rutabaga
- 1 Large Egg
- 2 ounces of Shredded Cheese
- 2 tablespoons of Bacon Grease
- Onion Powder
- Granulated Garlic
- Salt
- Pepper

Directions

1. Peel and quarter your rutabaga. Shred 4 ounces of rutabaga. Combine your cheese and egg with rutabaga. Mix well. Heat your bacon grease in your skillet. Add your mixture. Cook for a few minutes is turning it once. Serve!

Nutritional Value

231 Calories.
8 grams of Protein.
6 grams of Carbs.
20 grams of Fat.

135. Kale & Bacon Chips

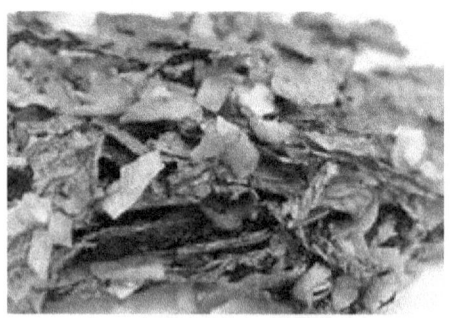

Ingredients

- One bunch of Kale
- Two tablespoons of Butter
- 1/4 cup of Bacon Grease
- Two teaspoons of Salt
- Garlic Powder

Directions

1. Preheat your oven to approximately 300 degrees. Remove leaves from kale. Tear kale into smaller bit sized pieces. Wash and dry thoroughly. Add your butter to bacon grease and warm until in a liquid state. Add in your salt and stir.

2. Put kale in a gallon sized Ziploc bag. Add your melted butter and bacon grease mixture. Don't completely seal the bag. You have to be able to shake kale leaves around so they can get completely coated. You want the leaves bright green. No dry leaves.

3. Pour your bag onto your cookie sheet. Make sure leaves are all in a single layer and completely coated. Sprinkle with your garlic powder. Bake approximately 20 to 25 minutes until the leaves turn dark green and get crispy but not burnt. Serve!

Nutritional Value

62 Calories.
One gram of Protein.
1 gram of Carbs.
6 grams of Fat.

136. Sautéed Cauliflower

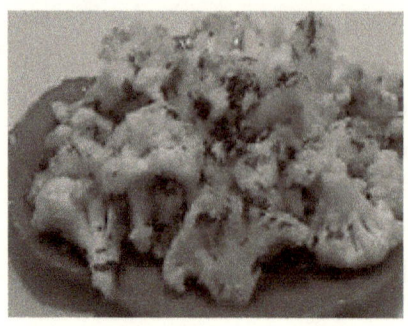

Ingredients

- 9 ounces of Cauliflower
- 1 tablespoon of Bacon Grease
- Salt
- Pepper

Directions

1. Boil your cauliflower for approximately 5 to 10 minutes. Squeeze any liquid out of your cauliflower using your potato ricer. Fry it in you are bacon grease. Season with salt and pepper when you're almost finished cooking. Serve!

137. Sautéed Mushrooms

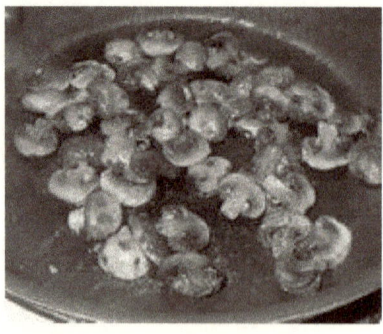

Serving size: This recipe yields 2 servings.

Ingredients

- 10 ounces of White Button Mushrooms
- 3 tablespoons of Bacon Grease
- One teaspoon of Parmesan Cheese
- Garlic
- Salt
- Pepper

Directions

1. Slice your mushrooms. Cook your mushrooms with bacon grease in your skillet. Season with your garlic powder, pepper, and salt. Grate your Parmesan cheese onto your mushrooms. Serve!

Nutritional Value

185 Calories.
4 grams of Protein.
4 grams of Carbs.
17 grams of Fat.

138. Bacon Wrapped Smokies

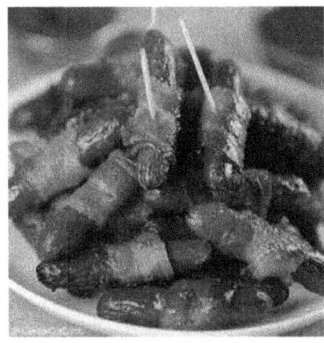

Ingredients

- 45 Smokies / Cocktail Wieners

- 10 slices of Bacon
- 45 Toothpicks

Directions

1. Cut your bacon into 3 or 4 strips. Wrap each of your wieners with a slice of bacon and spear it with one toothpick. Cook at 400 degrees until done. Finish them off with your broiler.

139. Beef and Bacon Heart Appetizer Rolls

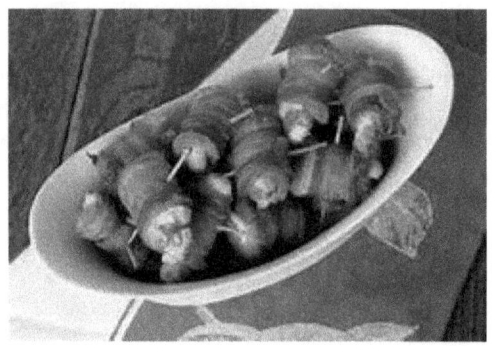

Ingredients

- ¼ tsp. Dried chili flakes
- ¼ tsp. Dried parsley
- ¼ tsp. Garlic powder
- ½ tsp. Celtic Sea Salt
- 12 Organic Uncured Bacon Slices
- 12 ounce Pastured Beef Heart meat, cut into 1 inch thick pieces

Directions

1. Combine salt and all the seasonings together. Sprinkle the seasoning mixture on the pastured beef heart meat. Wrap bacon around the flesh and use the toothpick to secure it.

2. Put the rolls on a broiler pan and set the grill on high cook until crispy and brown for about ten minutes. Serve with homemade mayonnaise mixed with hot sauce.

Nutritional Value

Calories 124
Fat 7g
Carbohydrates 0g
Protein 14g

140. Choco-Vanilla-Strawberries Fat Bombs

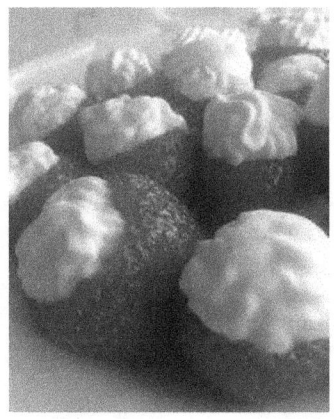

Ingredients

- Two tablespoons Cocoa Powder
- 2 tablespoon Erythritol
- 25 drops Liquid Stevia
- 1 teaspoon Vanilla Extract
- Two medium Strawberries
- 1/2 c. Butter
- 1/2 c. Coconut Oil
- 1/2 c. Sour Cream
- 1/2 c. Cream Cheese

Directions

1. Divide the mixture between 3 bowls. Add vanilla to one, cocoa powder to another and strawberries to the last bowl.

2. Pour the Choco mixture into fat bomb mold, place in the freezer for 30 min. Do the same thing with fruit and vanilla. Freeze for at least 1 hour.

Nutritional Value

Calories 102
Fats 10.9
Carbohydrates 0.4g
Protein 0.6g

141. Keto Flaxseed Tortilla Chips

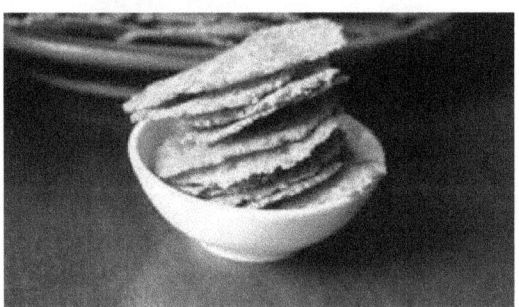

Ingredients

- Tortilla Chips
- 3 tablespoon Absorbed Oil
- 6 Flaxseed Tortillas
- Salt and Pepper to Taste

Optional Toppings

- Sour Cream

- Diced Jalapeno Shredded Cheese Salsa

Directions

1. Cut the tortillas into six parts. Preheat your deep fryer. Lay out 4 to 6 pieces of tortillas at a time. Fry for about one to two minutes then turn. Fry for another one to two minutes and cook the other side.

2. Take it out from the fryer and place on paper towel to cool down. Add pepper and salt to season. Top with your preferred toppings. Serve.

Nutritional Value

Calories 27
Fats 0.04g
Carbohydrates 0.04g
Protein 0.9g

142. Tasty Keto Hotdog Muffins

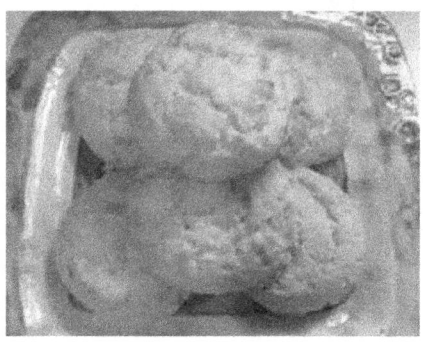

Ingredients

- One tablespoon Psyllium Husk Powder
- 3 tablespoon Swerve Sweetener
- One large Egg

- Ten little hotdogs (or 3 hot dogs)
- 1/2 c. Blanched Almond Flour
- 1/2 c. Flaxseed Meal
- 1/3 c. Sour Cream
- 1/4 teaspoon Salt
- 1/4 teaspoon Baking Powder
- 1/4 c. melted Butter
- 1/4 c. Coconut Milk

Directions

1. Preheat your oven to 375 degrees Fahrenheit. Combine the dry ingredients in a bowl. Add sour cream, butter, egg, milk and coconut milk and mix well. Divide the mixture into 20 greased mini-muffin slots. Slice the hot dogs and insert in the middle of each bread. Bake for 12 minutes and boil for one to two minutes until lightly brown on top.

2. Push the pieces of hot dog back into the muffin in case they rose with the batter. Cool the cupcakes in the tray for a few minutes then transfer it to the wire rack. You can also mix ketchup, chili paste, and mayonnaise together to make a sweet and spicy dip sauce.

Nutritional Value

Calories 79
Fats 6.8g
Carbohydrates 0.7g
Protein 2.4

143. Keto Flaxseed Cheeseburger Muffins

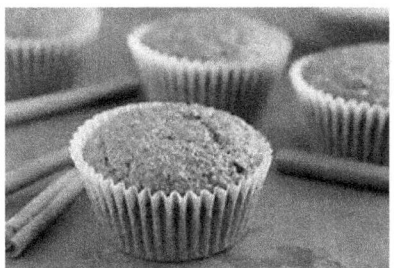

Ingredients

- Cheeseburger Muffin Buns
- 1 teaspoon Baking Powder
- Two large Eggs
- 1/2 c. Blanched Almond Flour
- 1/2 c. Flaxseed Meal
- 1/2 teaspoon Salt
- 1/4 teaspoon Pepper
- 1/4 c. Sour Cream
- Hamburger Filling
- 16-ounce Ground Beef
- Two tablespoon Tomato Paste
- Salt and Pepper to Taste
- 1/2 c. Cheddar Cheese
- 18 slices Baby Dill Pickles
- 2 tablespoon Mustard
- Two tablespoon Reduced Sugar Ketchup

Directions

1. In a hot pan, cook the ground beef with seasonings. Turn off the pot when seared. Combine the dry ingredients together for the muffins and preheat the oven to 350 degrees Fahrenheit. Then mix the wet and dry ingredients.

2. Divide the mixture into the silicone muffin cups. Create a space in the muffin for the ground beef. Then, add the ground beef

mixture in each muffin. Bake until browned on the outside or for 15 to 20 minutes.

3. Bake it out of the oven and top it with cheese, broil for another 1 to 3 minutes. Allow it to cool down for 5 to 10 minutes. Take it out of the silicone muffin cups and add your favorite toppings. Serve.

Nutritional Value

Calories 246
Fats 18.6g
Carbohydrates 1.9g
Protein 14.2g

144. Keto Churros in a Mug

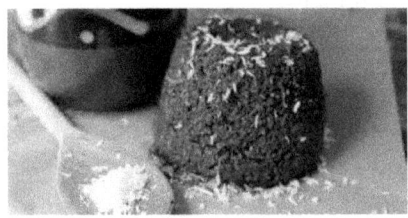

Ingredients for the Base

- 1 Egg
- One tablespoon Erythritol
- 1/2 teaspoon Baking Powder
- 2 tablespoon Almond Flour
- 2 tablespoon Butter
- 7 Drops Stevia

Ingredients for the Flavor

- 2 tablespoon Almond Flour
- 1/4 Teaspoon Cinnamon

- 1/4 teaspoon Nutmeg
- 1/4 teaspoon Vanilla
- 1/8 teaspoon Ginger
- 1/8 teaspoon Allspice

Directions

1. Combine all the ingredients together in the mug. Set your microwave in high and microwave for 60 seconds.

2. To transfer the churros into the serving plate, turn the cup upside down and bang it against a plate. Top with whipped cream and sprinkle erythritol and cinnamon.

Nutritional Value

Calories 437
Fats 4g
Carbohydrates 4g
Protein 12g

145. Easy to Do Keto Caprese Salad

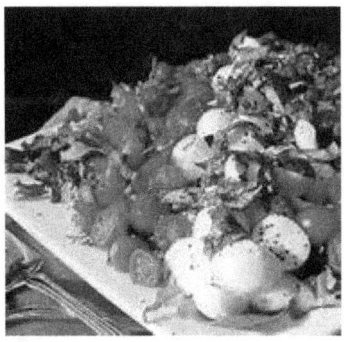

Ingredients

- 1 Fresh Tomato
- 1/4 c. chopped Fresh Basil

- 3 tablespoon Olive Oil
- 6-ounce Fresh Mozzarella Cheese
- Fresh Cracked Black Pepper
- Kosher Salt

Directions

1. Place the chopped basil leaves in a food processor and add two tablespoon olive oil and process until you got a paste like a mixture.

2. Slice the tomato into six slices. Cut the mozzarella, cheese into 1-ounce slices. Arrange Caprice salad by layering tomato, mozzarella and the basil paste. Add pepper, extra olive oil and salt.

Nutritional Value

Calories 405
Fats 36g
Carbohydrates 3.5g
Protein 15.5g

146. Cheesy Keto Broccoli Biscuits

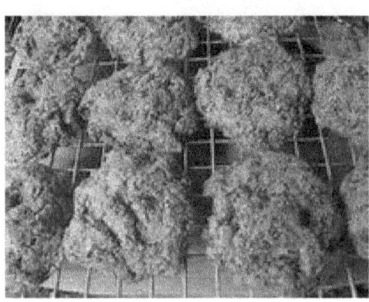

Ingredients

- 1 1/2 C. Almond Flour

- 1/2 teaspoon Apple Cider Vinegar
- One teaspoon Garlic Powder
- 1/2 teaspoon Baking Soda
- One teaspoon Paprika
- 1/2 teaspoon Pepper
- 1 teaspoon Salt
- 1/4 C. melted Coconut Oil
- 2 C. Cheddar Cheese
- 2 Large Eggs
- 4 C. Raw Broccoli Florets

Directions

1. Pre-heat your oven to 375 degrees Fahrenheit. Combine the spices and almond flour together, then add vinegar, coconut oil, and eggs. Mix thoroughly until dough forms. Combine your broccoli and shredded cheese in the flour mixture and mix well.

2. Create 12 patties from your dough and place them on your Silpat. Bake the biscuits for 12 to 15 minutes and take it out from the oven once done. Fix the shape to make it look like a cookie, then return the pan to the oven and bake for five minutes

3. Set your oven to broil and cook for 4 to 5 minutes more. Allow it to cool down for 3 to 4 mins. Then remove from the Silpat and enable it to cool down for 5 to 10 mins. On a cookie sheet.

Nutritional Value

Calories 163
Fats 14.3g
Carbohydrates 2g
Protein 6.8g

147. Pumpkin and Pistachio Choco Muffins

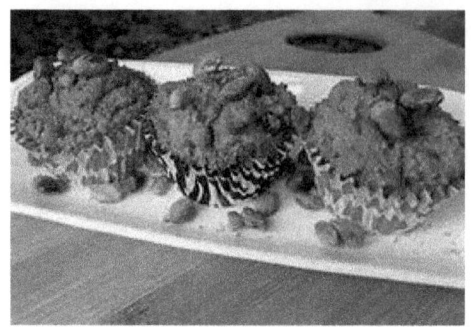

Ingredients

- 1 1/2 C. Almond Flour
- 1 1/2 teaspoon Cinnamon
- 1/2 C. Erythritol
- 1/2 C. Pistachios (Pre-salted)
- 1/2 C. Pumpkin Puree
- 1/2 teaspoon Apple Cider Vinegar
- 1/2 teaspoon Baking Soda
- 1/2 teaspoon Cloves
- 1/2 teaspoon Ginger
- 1/2 teaspoon Nutmeg
- 1/4 C. Coconut Oil
- 2 Large Eggs
- 2 teaspoon Quality Vanilla
- 3 Choco Perfection Dark Bars

Directions

1. Preheat oven to 325F. Combine Baking Soda, Almond Flour, Spices, and Erythritol. Mix well. In a separate mixing bowl, combine Pumpkin Puree, Large Eggs, Apple Cider Vinegar, Vanilla, and Coconut Oil. You can start by adding only 1/2 of the liquid into the dry. Continue mixing until thoroughly combined.

2. Cut the Choco Perfection Bars. Insert the pistachios and chocolate to the batter and fold them in. Divide the mixture

between 8 Cupcake Liners. Bake until golden brown or for 25-30 minutes

Nutritional Value

Calories 231
Fats 21.5g
Carbohydrates 4g
Protein 6.6g

148. Keto Spice Fritters with Lemon and Cinnamon

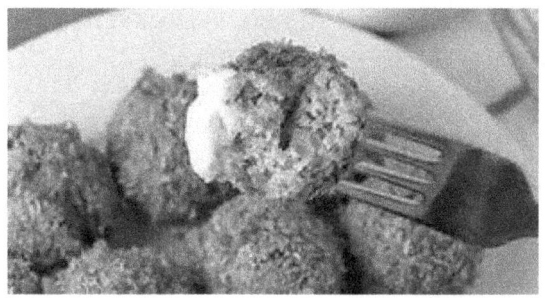

Ingredients

- Spicy Fritters
- 1 Large Egg
- One teaspoon Baking Powder
- 1/2 c. Almond Flour
- 1/2 teaspoon Xanthan Gum
- 2 Cups Fat of Your Choice (For Frying)
- 3 tablespoon Erythritol
- Three tablespoons Powdered Erythritol
- Juice of 1/4 Lemon
- Lemon Glaze
- Zest of 1/2 Lemon

Directions

1. Combine all the dry ingredients together and mix well. Add egg and mix well to form the sticky dough. Heat oil on the stove up to 375 degrees Fahrenheit, if you don't have a thermometer to measure the temperature, you can drop a small piece of dough to check if the oil is hot enough. The dough will fry if it is ready.

2. Drop four dough balls at a time. Fry until brown then turn on the other side and cook again until brown. Remove the cooked dough and place on paper towels, and continue to fry the remaining dough. Combine erythritol and lemon juice in a small bowl mix until a smooth icing is formed. Before serving the fritters dip it first in the icing and serving.

Nutritional Value

Calories 50
Fats 4.6g
Carbohydrates 0.7g
Protein 1.7g

149. Cheese Flavored Keto Chips

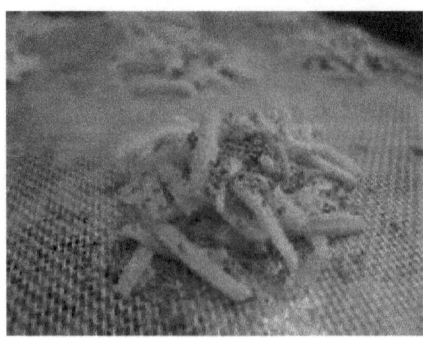

Ingredients

- 1 1/2 c. Cheddar Cheese

- Three tablespoon Ground Flaxseed Meal
- Seasonings of Your Choice

Directions

1. Pre-heat the oven to 425 degrees Fahrenheit. Make two tablespoon mounds of cheddar cheese on a non-stick silicone pad. Sprinkle a pinch of flaxseed on each chip until you used up all the flaxseed. Distribute it evenly.

2. Add your preferred seasonings to each dip. Bake for ten minutes and take it out of the oven once done. Cool and transfer them to a serving plate. Serve.

Nutritional Value

Calories 54
Fats 5.6g
Carbohydrates 0.5g
Protein 3.9g

150. Sweet Keto Choco Cake in a Mug

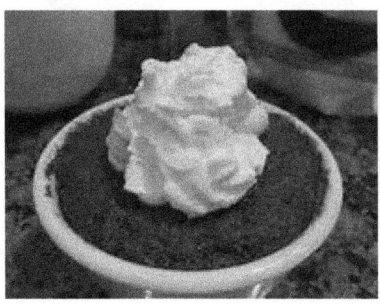

Ingredients

- 1 1/2 tablespoon Erythritol or Splenda
- 1 Large Egg
- Two tablespoon Salted Butter

- Two tablespoons Unsweetened Cocoa Powder
- Two teaspoons Coconut Flour

Directions

1. Microwave the butter for 25 seconds until it melts. Add the other ingredients into the batter and mix well. Microwave again for another 60 to 75 seconds. As the topping, you can whip some heavy cream.

Nutritional Value

Calories 197
Fats 19g
Carbohydrates 2.6g
Protein 6g

151. Pumpkin Flaxseed Keto Cookies with Almond Butter Icing

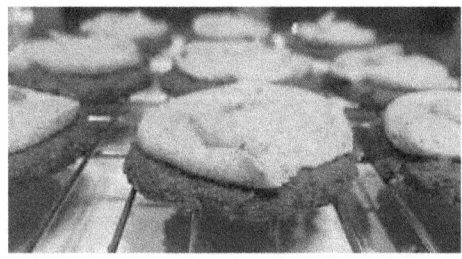

Ingredients for the Cookies

- 1 c. Blanched Almond Flour
- 1 Large Egg
- One teaspoon Vanilla Extract
- One teaspoon Cinnamon
- 1/2 c. Flaxseed Meal
- 1/2 c. Pumpkin Puree
- 1/2 teaspoon Nutmeg

- 1/4 c. Salted Butter
- 1/4 c. Coconut Oil
- 1/4 c. Erythritol
- 1/4 teaspoon Fresh Ground Clove

Ingredients for the Icing

- Two tablespoons Erythritol
- 1 tablespoon Heavy Cream
- One teaspoon Vanilla Extract
- 1/4 c. Butter
- 1/4 c. Cream Cheese
- 1/4 c. Almond Butter

Directions

1. Pre-heat the oven to 350 degrees Fahrenheit. Combine the flaxseed meal, spices, almond flour and erythritol together. Microwave for 30 seconds the coconut oil and butter to melt it. Combine the dry ingredients and the butter/coconut oil mixture. Add the egg and pumpkin puree and mix well. Make balls out of the dough and lay them on the baking sheet. Press the dough down and place them in the oven. Cook for 12 to 15 mins.

2. In making the icing, combine all the ingredients using a fork and mix using a hand blender until fluffy. Remove from the oven and allow them to cool down and store them in the fridge overnight. You might notice that it is a little bit soggy-ish when you take them out of the oven, but they will harden when placed in the fridge. Place the icing in a Ziploc bag, make a small cut in the corner and ice the cookies.

Nutritional Value

Calories 132
Fats 13g

Carbohydrates 1.3g
Protein 2.8g

152. Ketogenic Chocolate Coconut Cookies

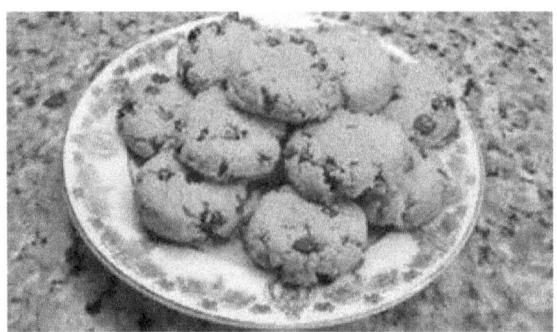

Serving size: This recipe yields 20 servings.

Ingredients

- 1 cup almond flour
- Two eggs (unchilled)
- ½ tsp. baking powder
- 1/3 cup unsweet shredded coconut
- ¼ cup cocoa powder
- ¼ cup coconut oil
- 3 tbsp. coconut flour
- 1/3 cup erythritol
- ¼ tsp. salt
- One tsp. Vanilla extract

Directions

1. Preheat your oven to 350 degrees. While your oven preheats, line a large cookie sheet with parchment paper. In a medium sized mixing bowl, combine your dry ingredients and mix well using your hand mixer.

2. In a separate bowl, combine all of your wet ingredients together and mix well using your hand mixer. Slowly add your wet ingredient mixture to your dry ingredient mixture while mixing until all of your ingredients are combined.

3. Now, break off small pieces of your dough and roll them into little cookie balls. You should be able to get around 20 balls out of your bowl of dough. Set each of your cookie balls onto your parchment covered sheet. Bake your cookies in your preheated oven for 15 to 20 minutes or until cooked through.

Nutrition Per Serving

Calories 77
Fat 6.8g
Protein 2.2g
Carbs 2.5g
Sugar 0g
Fiber 1.5g

153. Ketogenic Nut Butter Cookies

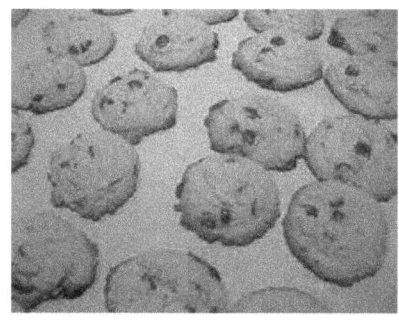

Serving size: This recipe yields 10 servings.

Ingredients

- 1 egg
- 8.8oz. almond butter

- ¼ tsp. salted butter
- ¼ cup powdered erythritol
- ¼ cup raw coconut butter

Directions

1. Preheat your oven to 320 degrees. While your oven preheats, cover a large cookie sheet with parchment paper. Melt your almond butter in a double boiler or a bowl inside a saucepan of hot water.

2. Once your almond butter has melted remove your bowl from the pan and take the pan off your heat. Now, add in your salt, erythritol, and egg to the bowl of melted almond butter. With a silicone spatula, fold your ingredients together until fully mixed.

3. Once your ingredients are well mixed, break your dough into ten pieces. Roll each piece between your hands to make balls of dough. Set each ball of dough onto your parchment paper covered cookie tray. Gently flatten your cookies using the palm of your hand or a fork. Bake your cookies for 12 minutes in your preheated oven until browned.

Nutrition Per Serving

Calories 235
Fat 22g
Protein 5g
Carbs 11g
Sugar 1g
Fiber 4g

154. Ketogenic Strawberry Thumbprint Cookies

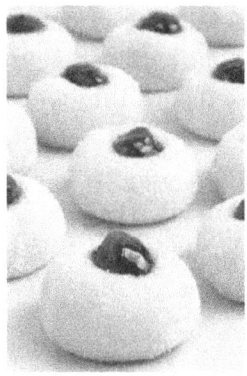

Serving size: This recipe yields 16 servings.

Ingredients

- 2 tbsp. coconut flour
- 1 cup almond flour
- ½ tsp. baking powder
- 1 tbsp. shredded coconut
- 2 tbsp. sugar-free strawberry jam
- 2 eggs
- 4 tbsp. coconut oil
- ½ cup Erythritol
- ½ tsp. salt
- ¼ tsp. cinnamon
- ½ tsp. almond extract
- ½ tsp. vanilla extract

Directions

1. Preheat your oven to 350 degrees. While your oven preheats, cover a large cookie sheet with parchment paper. In a large mixing bowl use a whisk to mix all of your dry ingredients. Once well mixed, make a well in the center of your dry ingredients and add in your wet ingredients. Use your whisk again to combine the dry and wet ingredients together.

2. Once well mixed, break your dough into 16 pieces and roll each one into a ball. Set your balls of dough on the parchment covered cookie sheet and used your thumb to press a thumbprint in the center of each cookie. Set your cookies out on a cookie rack to cool completely. Once your cookies are cooled, add a small amount of your strawberry jam into each thumbprint and sprinkle with your coconut.

Nutrition Per Serving

Calories 95
Fat 9g
Protein 2g
Carbs 4g
Sugar 0g
Fiber 3g

155. Ketogenic Coconut Macaroon Cookies

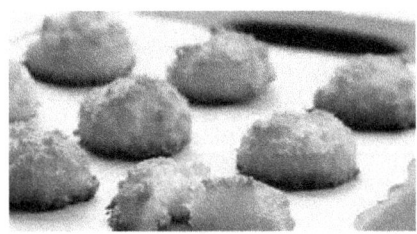

Serving size: This recipe yields 12 servings.

Ingredients

- 1 cup unsweetened shredded coconut
- One egg white
- One dash salt
- 2 tbsp. coconut oil
- ¼ cup erythritol
- ½ tsp. almond extract

Directions

1. Preheat your oven to 350 degrees. While your oven preheats, cover a large cookie sheet with parchment paper. Spread your coconut out onto the journal covered cookie sheet. When your oven comes to heat, toast the coconut until browned. Once cooked, take your coconut out of the oven and let it cool completely.

2. Now in a large mixing bowl, use a hand mixer to beat your egg white until it doubles in size and add your salt and erythritol as you are still mixing. Pour in your almond extract and your toasted, cooled coconut and mix thoroughly. Use your hands to roll 12 balls out of your dough and lay them out on your parchment covered cookie sheet. Bake your macaroons for around 15 minutes or until golden brown.

Nutrition Per Serving

Calories 88
Fat 8g
Protein 1g
Carbs 4g
Sugar 1g
Fiber 2g

156. Ketogenic Pumpkin Spice Cookies

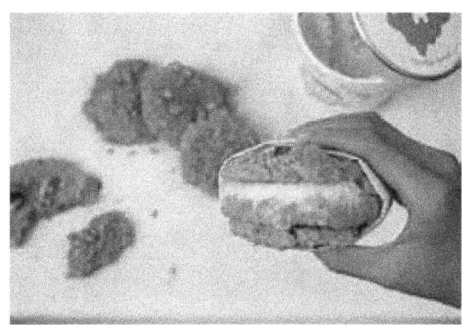

Serving size: This recipe yields 15 servings.

Ingredients

- 1 ½ cup almond flour
- ½ tsp. baking powder
- 1 egg
- ½ cup pumpkin puree
- ¼ cup salted butter
- One tsp. vanilla extract
- ¼ cup erythritol
- 25 drops liquid Stevia
- Two extra drops of erythritol
- One tsp. Pumpkin pie spice

Directions

1. Preheat your oven to 350 degrees. While your oven preheats, cover a large cookie sheet with parchment paper. In a large mixing bowl, combine your baking powder, flour, and ¼ cup erythritol. Stir together with a silicone spatula.

2. In a clean microwave-safe bowl, combine your pumpkin puree, butter, vanilla, and liquid Stevia. Add in your microwaved ingredients into your dry ingredients. Mix well using your silicone spatula until you get a sticky dough.

3. Use a teaspoon to scoop your dough into 15 servings and use your hands to roll each serving into a ball. Set the cookie balls onto your parchment paper and use your palm to flatten each one gently.

4. Put your cookies in the oven to bake for 12 minutes. As your cookies bake, add your two drops of erythritol to your pumpkin pie spice and use your food processor to mix. When your cookies

have cooked through, sprinkle the top of each with your pumpkin pie spice mixture out of the food processor.

Nutrition Per Serving

Calories 75
Fat 7g
Protein 2g
Carbs 3g
Sugar 1g
Fiber 2g

157. Ketogenic Chocolate Chip Cookies

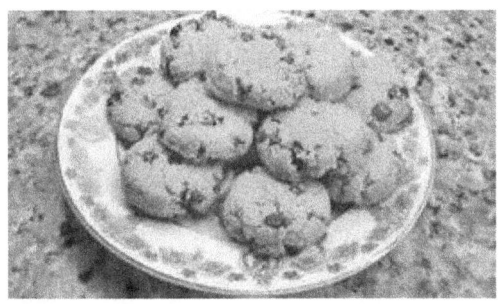

Serving size: This recipe yields 16 servings.

Ingredients

- 1 cup almond flour
- 2 tbsp. coconut flour
- ½ tsp. baking powder
- 2 tbsp. psyllium husk powder
- 3 tbsp. whey protein
- 1 egg
- 1 cup dark chocolate chips
- 8 tbsp. room temperature unsalted butter
- ¼ cup erythritol
- Two tsp. vanilla extract

- 10 drops liquid Stevia

Directions

1. Preheat your oven to 350 degrees. While your oven preheats, cover a large cookie sheet with parchment paper. In a large mixing bowl, combine your coconut flour, almond meal, baking powder, psyllium husk powder, and whey protein. Stir with a silicone spatula to combine your ingredients.

2. Now, in a clean medium-sized mixing bowl, use your hand mixer to mix the butter for just a couple of minutes until it pales. Add in 10 drops of your liquid Stevia and ¼ cup of erythritol and mix again to combine.

3. Add your vanilla extract and egg into the butter bowl and mix again until you get a smooth batter. Once your butter is smooth, use a sieve to sift your dry ingredients over the butter ingredients. Use your hand mixer again to combine your ingredients fully.

4. Set your hand mixer down and use your spatula to fold in your dark chocolate chips evenly. Once your chocolate chips are folded in, pull off small pieces of dough and roll them into cookie balls. You should get 16 cookies.

5. When your cookie balls are laid out on your cookie sheet, use your palm or the bottom of a drinking glass to flatten your cookies gently. Bake your cookies for between 12 and 15 minutes until done.

Nutrition Per Serving

Calories 162
Fat 12g
Protein 3g
Carbs 13g

Sugar 6g
Fiber 3g

158. Ketogenic Peanut Butter Chocolate Cookies

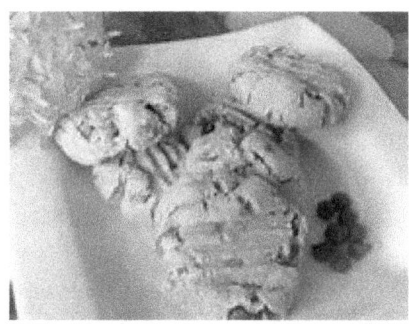

Serving size: This recipe yields 20 servings.

Ingredients

- 2 ½ cups almond flour
- 1 ½ tsp. baking soda
- 1 ½ tsp. baking powder
- ½ tsp. salt
- 3 tbsp. no sugar added maple syrup
- ½ cup natural creamy peanut butter
- 20 Hershey's dark chocolate minis
- 1 tbsp. vanilla extract
- ¼ cup coconut oil
- ¼ cup erythritol

Directions

1. In a large mixing bowl, combine ¼ cup coconut oil, ½ cup peanut butter, 1 tbsp. Vanilla extract, and 3 tbsp. Maple syrup. Use your hand mixer to mix these ingredients together until you get a smooth batter.

2. In a second mixing bowl, combine 1 ½ tsp. Baking powder, 2 ½ cups almond flour, ½ tsp. Salt, and ¼ cup erythritol. Stir these ingredients together with a silicone spatula to combine.

3. Once well mixed, use a sieve to sprinkle your dry ingredients over your batter. Use your mixer to combine all of the ingredients in your bowl until you get a rough dough.

4. Now, use your hands to roll the dough into a big round ball and wrap it tightly in a sheet of plastic wrap. Put your wrapped dough in the refrigerator and let sit for 30 minutes.

5. Preheat your oven to 350 degrees while your dough chills. Unwrap your 20 mini dark chocolate pieces and then cover a large cookie sheet with parchment paper.

6. When your dough is chilled, take it out of the oven and divide it into 20 pieces. Wrap each piece of dough around a single dark chocolate mini piece. Make sure that the chocolate is completely surrounded by dough when folding your cookies. Bake your cookies for 15 minutes or until thoroughly cooked and allow to cool before eating.

Nutrition Per Serving

Calories 262
Fat 23g
Protein 3g
Carbs 15g
Sugar 7g
Fiber 5g

159. Ketogenic Snickerdoodles

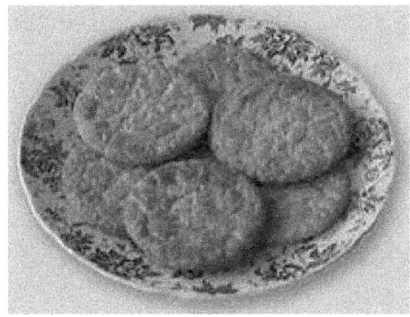

Serving size: This recipe yields 14 servings.

Ingredients

- 2 cups almond flour
- ¼ tsp. baking soda
- ¼ cup maple syrup
- ¼ cup coconut oil
- 1 tbsp. vanilla
- 7 drops liquid Stevia
- Dash of salt
- 2 tbsp. cinnamon
- 2 tbsp. erythritol

Directions

1. Preheat your oven to 350 degrees. While your oven preheats, cover a large cookie sheet with parchment paper. In a large mixing bowl, combine 1 tbsp. Vanilla, ¼ cup melted coconut oil, 7 drops liquid Stevia and ¼ cup maple syrup. Use a silicone spatula to stir your ingredients together.

2. In another bowl, combine ¼ tsp. Baking soda, a dash of salt, and 2 cups almond flour. Mix well and then slowly add in your wet ingredients to your dry. Mix until you get a cookie dough. Now, use a small bowl to combine your 2 tbsp. Erythritol and 2 tbsp. cinnamon. Mix these together. Use your hands to roll your cookie

dough into 14 small balls and roll each ball in your cinnamon mixture to cover it completely.

3. Set out your covered cookie balls on your parchment covered cookie sheet and use the palm of your hand of the bottom of glass to flatten them gently. Bake your cookies for 10 minutes and then pull them out of the oven to cool.

Nutrition Per Serving

Calories 132
Fat 12.4g
Protein 3.4g
Carbs 4.2g
Sugar 5.5g
Fiber 2.2g

160. Ketogenic Coffee Time Cookies

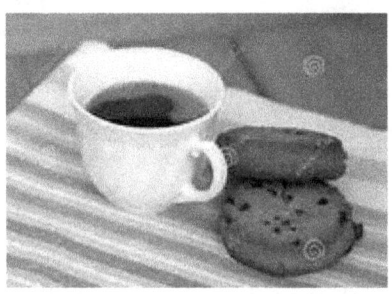

Serving size: This recipe yields 10 servings.

Ingredients

- 1 ½ cups almond flour
- ½ tsp. baking soda
- ½ tsp. salt
- ½ cup room temperature unsalted butter
- 1 tbsp. And one tsp. Instant coffee grounds

- 2 eggs
- 1/3 cup erythritol
- 17 drops liquid Stevia
- 1 ½ tsp. vanilla extract
- ¼ tsp. cinnamon

Directions

1. While your oven preheats, cover a large cookie tray with parchment paper. In a large mixing bowl, combine your 1 ½ cups almond flour, ½ tsp. Baking soda, ½ tsp. salt, coffee grounds, and ¼ tsp. cinnamon. Stir with a silicone spatula to mix thoroughly.

2. Using two small bowls or short drinking glasses, crack your eggs, separating your whites and yolks. Now, add your butter to a clean bowl and whip it to a creamy consistency using your hand mixer. Once it's finished beating, add in 1/3 cup erythritol and whip again using your hand mixer. This time you want to hit until your butter turns almost white.

3. When your butter is almost white, add your egg yolks and mix again until combined. Once combined, add half of your dry ingredients into your butter mixture and whip.

4. When half your dry ingredients are thoroughly mixed in to your wet, add 17 drops of liquid Stevia and 1 ½ tsp. Vanilla extract along with the rest of your dry ingredients and then mix again until well combined.

5. Clean your mixer and then use it to whip your egg whites until you have stiff peaks and then fold them into your dough. Tear your dough into ten pieces, roll into cookies and set on your baking sheet. Press down gently to flatten and then bake in your preheated oven for 12 minutes or until browned.

Nutrition Per Serving

Calories 167
Fat 17.1g
Protein 3.9g
Carbs 2.8g
Sugar 7.4g
Fiber 1.4g

Don't forget to share your thoughts on this book by leaving a review on Amazon.com. It takes just a few seconds.

Are You ALWAYS Hungry When You Try to Lose Weight?

Discover How to STOP Starving Yourself & Lose Weight FASTER By Eating MORE Food!

For this month only, you can get Kayla's best-selling & most popular book absolutely free – *The Ultimate Guide to Healthy Eating & Losing Weight Without Starving Yourself!*

Get Your FREE Copy Here:
TopFitnessAdvice.com/Book

Discover how you can **start eating MORE food** and see weight loss results faster than ever before. Learn about the 10 most powerful fat-burning foods and how they boost the rate that your body burns fat. And last but not least, finally put an end to your emotional or "bored" eating habits. With this book, readers were able to significantly improve their weight loss results. So, it's highly recommended that you get this book, especially while it's free!

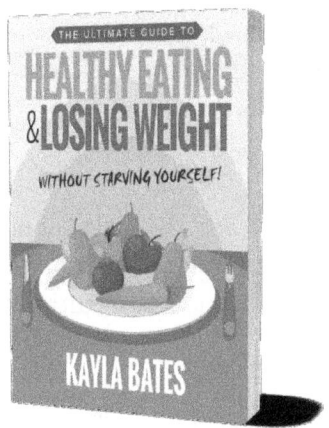

Get Your FREE Copy Here:
TopFitnessAdvice.com/Book

Conclusion

Thank you again for purchasing this book!

I hope this book was able to help you to learn Ketogenic diet.

Finding healthy and easy recipes is one of the biggest challenges you'll face when on a Ketogenic Diet. In our modern lives, we rarely have time to cook for ourselves every single day. Between work, bringing kids to practice, and cleaning up around the house, cooking healthy meals is usually the first thing to suffer.

The book is designed to make finding the perfect ketogenic diet recipe easy. The book is divided into nine parts:

Why should you go on a ketogenic diet-benefits and drawbacks of ketogenic diet:

- Effects of the ketogenic diet
- Getting started with the ketogenic diet
- Ketogenic diet plan
- Making the ketogenic diet work
- Low carb living tips for weight loss
- Tips for success on the ketogenic diet
- Low carb diet myths debunked
- Ketogenic diet recipes

Under each section you will get a new idea about the ketogenic diet.
Now is the time to bring your theoretical cooking knowledge into practice and get cooking some delicious and healthy ketogenic meals for your family.

So, what are you waiting for, get cooking right away.

Enjoying this book?

Check out my other best sellers!

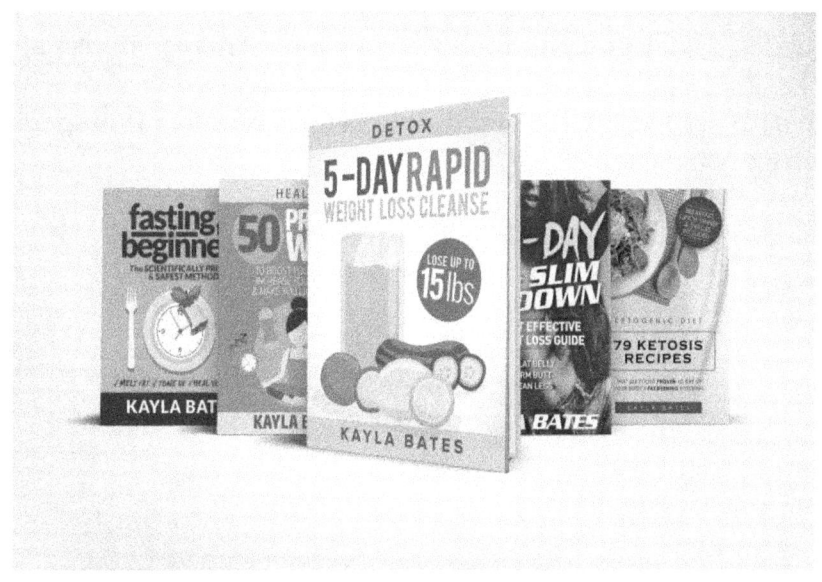

Get your next book on sale here:

TopFitnessAdvice.com/go/Kayla

Final Words

I would like to thank you for purchasing my book and I hope I have been able to help you and educate you on something new.

If you have enjoyed this book and would like to share your positive thoughts, could you please take 30 seconds of your time to go back and give me a review on my Amazon book page.

I greatly appreciate seeing these reviews because it helps me share my hard work.

You can leave me a review on Amazon.com.

Again, thank you and I wish you all the best!

www.ingramcontent.com/pod-product-compliance
Lightning Source LLC
Chambersburg PA
CBHW031144020426
42333CB00013B/502